Research Approaches in Primary Care

Edited
Andrew Wilson
Martin Williams
and
Beverley Hancock

Foreword by
Mike Pringle

Radcliffe Medical Press

©2000 Trent Focus Group

Radcliffe Medical Press Ltd
18 Marcham Road, Abingdon, Oxon OX14 1AA

All rights reserved. No part of this publication may be reproduced, stored in a retrieval system or transmitted, in any form or by any means, electronic, mechanical, photocopying, recording or otherwise, without the prior permission of the copyright owner.

British Library Cataloguing in Publication Data

A catalogue record for this book is available from the British Library.

ISBN 1 85775 392 5

Typeset by Advance Typesetting Ltd, Oxfordshire
Printed and bound by TJ International Ltd, Padstow, Cornwall

Contents

Foreword	vii
Volume editors	viii
List of contributors	ix
Introduction *Andrew Wilson*	1

1 An introduction to research methodology — 3
Beverley Hancock

Introduction	3
Identifying the research problem	4
Reviewing the literature	6
Methodology	7
Summary	19
Answers to exercises	20

2 Experimental designs — 23
Heather Wharrad

Introduction	23
Basic principles of experimental design	25
Research designs	36
Benefits and limitations of experimental research	44
Answers to exercises	47
References	51
Further reading	52
Self-completing glossary	52

3 Qualitative research — 55
Beverley Hancock

Introduction	55
The nature of qualitative research	56
Qualitative research designs	58
Methods of collecting qualitative data	62
Handling qualitative research data	66

	Analysing qualitative data	68
	Presenting the results of qualitative research	73
	Summary	75
	Answers to exercises	75
	References and further reading	76
4	**Surveys and questionnaires**	**77**
	Nigel Mathers, Nick Fox and Amanda Hunn	
	Introduction	77
	What is a survey?	77
	Methods of collecting survey data	81
	Sampling for surveys	84
	Questionnaire design	91
	Using questionnaires in postal surveys	102
	Data analysis	105
	Summary	106
	Answers to exercises	107
	Further reading	110
	Appendix 1: The Fog Index	111
5	**Using interviews in a research project**	**113**
	Nigel Mathers, Nick Fox and Amanda Hunn	
	Introduction	113
	Types of interview	114
	Interviewer tasks and skills	118
	Sources of error and bias in interviewing	120
	Preparing and conducting the interview	121
	Handling interview data	128
	Summary	132
	Answers to exercises	132
	References and further reading	134
	Further resources	134
6	**Data collection by observation**	**135**
	Nick Fox	
	Introduction	135
	Observation as a research method	136
	When and why should we use ethnographic methods?	138
	Observing in the field: finding a role	139
	Becoming an observer	140

Access	140
Methods of observation	143
Note-taking	144
Understanding and interpretation	145
Putting it into practice: the inside view	148
Validity and reliability in observational studies	149
Criticism of observational research	152
Conclusion	154
Answers to exercises	154
References	159
Further reading	159
Glossary	161
Index	173

Foreword

Research into primary care is under-developed, not just amongst general practitioners but also nurses and other health professionals. Primary care cannot be expected to move from the twilight into the spotlight without support. The welcome access for general practices and community trusts to Culyer research and development funding has started to redress the resource inequality between primary and secondary care. However, the greatest shortage has been in research skills, as those involved have not routinely been expected to undertake research in their training and, for many, research skills appear foreign and demanding.

The recognition of these realities led Trent Regional Health Authority – now the Trent Regional Office of the NHS Executive – to support the Trent Focus for the Promotion of Research and Development in Primary Health Care from 1995 onwards. The Focus has existed primarily to enhance the research skills of those working in primary care on a regional basis. It does this through offering education and support to those interested in research; buying specific research advice for those undertaking research; supporting research clubs; running a collaborating research practices scheme; and funding designated research practices which undertake original research.

Out of this work recognition emerged that some research issues came up time and again, and that the standard reference works do not cover them satisfactorily. Thus the idea for this series was born. These volumes synthesise current wisdom on how to successfully start in primary care research. They are not intended to provide definitive texts, nor to be used as the only source of knowledge. They will, however, cover most of the issues that a nascent researcher will encounter, and will inspire many to try their hand.

For the truth is this: research can be wonderfully stimulating, enriching our daily clinical work, and helping to improve care for future generations. However, like most areas of human activity, it is only worth doing if it is done well – and that requires skills, support, advice, insight and perseverance. Those who read and use these volumes will stand a better chance of doing good research, and should obtain real pleasure from it.

Professor Mike Pringle
Chairman
RCGP
October 1999

Volume editors

Dr Andrew Wilson
Trent Focus Regional Coordinator
University of Leicester

Martin Williams
Trent Focus Local Coordinator
De Montfort University

Beverley Hancock
Trent Focus Local Coordinator
Division of General Practice
University of Nottingham

List of contributors

Dr Nick Fox
Senior Lecturer
Institute of General Practice and
 Primary Care
University of Sheffield

Amanda Hunn
Trent Focus Local Coordinator
Institute of General Practice and
 Primary Care
University of Sheffield

Professor Nigel Mathers
Director
Institute of General Practice and
 Primary Care
University of Sheffield

Dr Heather Wharrad
Lecturer, Postgraduate Division
School of Nursing
University of Nottingham

Introduction

Andrew Wilson

Primary care is notable for the diversity of its research approaches. This is not surprising, given the range of unanswered questions that daily present themselves to practitioners, and the different scientific and philosophical backgrounds of practitioners themselves. Priorities for someone starting research in primary care are to gain an overview of the methods available, to be able to find an appropriate method to tackle their research question, and to be aware of when specialist advice is needed and where to find it. This volume aims to address these issues.

In Chapter 1, Beverley Hancock provides an overview of research methods in primary care. She emphasises that before choosing a method, the first step is to develop a researchable idea, whether it is presented as an aim, hypothesis or question. Next the literature should be reviewed to identify previous work and gaps in knowledge. After these steps have been undertaken, it is likely that strong pointers will be available to identify the most appropriate research method.

In Chapter 2, Heather Wharrad describes experimental designs, covering 'n of one', 'within group' and 'between group' designs, including a discussion of the advantages and disadvantages of the randomised controlled trial. She introduces key concepts such as bias, confounding, validity and generalisability, which will also be of use when considering non-experimental methodologies.

Chapter 3, also by Beverley Hancock, describes the particular contribution that can be made by qualitative methods, and the key features of four different types of approach (phenomenology, ethnography, ground theory and case study). Like the authors of the remaining chapters, she moves on from issues of design to discuss data collection, analysis and interpretation.

In Chapter 4, Nigel Mathers and colleagues discuss the place of surveys as a research design, and the choice of survey instruments, including a detailed discussion of questionnaires, probably the most frequently used instrument. They cover such essential areas as how to design questionnaires, the benefit of using previously validated instruments, and how to determine whether to administer them by post or interview.

In Chapter 5, the same team discuss interviews in more detail, from highly structured to in-depth approaches, including telephone interviews and focus group techniques. As they point out, many of the communication skills developed in clinical work are transferable to conducting research interviews, but there are important differences between them, not least the workload implications of transcribing and analysing qualitative interview data.

In the final chapter, Nick Fox describes the use of ethnographic observation, as well as discussing more generally how the concepts of validity and reliability can be applied to qualitative methods. As in other volumes, all chapters include exercises to encourage readers to check their understanding of the contents, and relate them to their own experience.

CHAPTER ONE

An introduction to research methodology

Beverley Hancock

Introduction

Research can be defined as a process of systematic investigation of a subject for the purpose of adding to the body of knowledge about that subject. Contained in that definition are three key points:

- research is a process: it is carried out in stages
- investigation is carried out systematically: the investigation is planned
- research is intended to add to the body of knowledge: the purpose of research is to inform.

The process of research is made up of a number of stages that the researcher must proceed through for the research project to be completed satisfactorily. The stages are listed in Box 1.1 below.

Box 1.1   The research process

1. Identification of the research problem.
2. Review of the literature.
3. Defining the methodology.
4. Access and ethical considerations.
5. Pilot study.
6. Data collection.
7. Data analysis (results).
8. Drawing conclusions (includes identification of limitations and recommendations for practice and/or further research).

The purpose of this chapter is to introduce the reader to the major features of the research process. The type of information that informs decisions about how to undertake a research project will be described and supported by examples from primary care research. Exercises will be used to reinforce the reader's understanding of the text. The chapter is intended for use by primary healthcare professionals with little or no previous research knowledge.

The aims of this chapter are:

1. To explore how research ideas start.
2. To introduce the reader to different types of research.
3. To explain the basics of research methodology.
4. To identify the first steps in designing a feasible research project.

The Trent Focus has produced a series of three volumes addressing different aspects of research. The Trent Focus series has been designed to take into account that readers may have a variety of reasons for wanting to develop their research knowledge. This chapter provides a basic introduction to the research process for primary healthcare staff with no previous research training. Readers who already have a basic knowledge of the research process may find the chapter useful for revision. The reader will be directed at appropriate points in the text to other volumes in the Trent Focus series for further information, but its selection will depend on the reader's individual motivation for wanting more information.

If you want to know more about how to implement research findings you may find it useful to read this chapter before moving onto the Trent Focus volume *Developing Research in Primary Care*: Chapter 6, 'Implementing research findings'.

If you intend to undertake a research project you may find it useful to read this chapter before moving on to the Trent Focus volume *Developing Research in Primary Care*: Chapter 1, 'Starting a research project and applying for funding'.

Identifying the research problem

Every research project starts with an idea. All of us, in our work and our lives in general, constantly come across situations about which we would like to know more, or which we would like to understand better. We wonder about phenomena that we come across and ask ourselves questions like:

'I wonder why this happens?'
'How could I stop this from happening?'
'I wonder if it happens anywhere else?'

We review our performance and wonder how we can improve it by asking questions like:

'How can I do this better?'
'Can I do this more quickly/less expensively/differently?'
'Are people satisfied with my performance?'

Turning these questions into a *researchable* idea is the first stage of the research process. Sometimes our original idea is too difficult to research because it would take too long to find out the answer or it would take too many resources. If this is the case, the original idea has to be narrowed down to a manageable focus. For example, we may want to know if we are doing a good job. This sounds reasonable. But whom do we ask in order to find out? And how do we define what is meant by 'a good job'. If we spend a long time with each of our patients they may think we're doing a marvellous job, but our managers might not be very happy if we are not seeing enough patients, or we spend a fortune on treating each patient.

Although identifying a researchable idea is theoretically the first stage of the research process, it is quite common for the idea to be modified as the researcher starts to plan the subsequent stages of the research process. As we shall see, the second stage of the process – reviewing the literature – clarifies whether the idea needs to be researched or whether the answers to our questions already exist. The third stage of the research process is defining the methodology. This is where the researcher plans how to conduct the investigation and at this stage it may become clear that the research focus is still too big to be manageable or that the people who would be needed to provide the information cannot be easily accessed.

Despite this it is a good idea, at an early stage, to try and identify a phrase that describes the focus of the research. The research idea or research problem as it is often described, can be stated as an *aim*, a *question* or a *hypothesis*. Indeed, it may take more than one aim, question or hypothesis to adequately describe the purpose of the intended research.

It is not the case that one type of research statement is better than another, but that some types of research are better described by using one rather than another. Research which is concerned with exploring or describing phenomena often uses aims or research questions to describe the research problem, whereas research concerned with testing out an idea frequently uses a hypothesis.

The important element common to any research problem is that it should be researchable. For example, the question 'what is a good doctor?' is not answerable because there is no single answer; different people and different groups would have varying ideas about what makes a good doctor. However, if the study sets out to investigate 'patients' perceptions of what they see as a good doctor', this is researchable because patients' perceptions can be investigated. The following rules should be observed in stating the research problem:

- an aim must be achievable
- a question must be answerable
- a hypothesis must be testable.

Exercise 1

It is frequently possible to describe a research problem by using an aim, a question or a hypothesis. For example, if we wanted to look at the types of mental-health problem most frequently seen in general practice settings we could state this as:

- **aim** – the aim of the research is to identify the mental-health problems most frequently encountered in general practice
- **question** – what mental-health problems are most frequently encountered in general practice?
- **hypothesis** – depression and anxiety are encountered more frequently than any other mental-health problems in general practice.

Write an aim, a question and a hypothesis for the following research problem: ***patient satisfaction with the appointments system.***

Reviewing the literature

As we saw in the previous section, every research project starts with an idea, something which the researcher is interested in knowing more about or is worried about – something that is perceived as a problem or as a knowledge gap which needs to be filled, but at the outset is often vague or too broad to be covered in one research project. More information is needed by the researcher in order for the problem to be refined to make it manageable and researchable. This is assisted by a review of existing literature.

Before embarking on any research project, the researcher should search and review existing literature. The literature review has several purposes as it provides answers to the following questions:

- what is currently known about the topic?
- what aspects of the topic lack sufficient information? (the gaps in the literature)
- what research has previously been done?
- what recommendations for further research have been previously made but not acted upon?
- what methods have previous researchers used to investigate the topic and were some methods better suited to the topic than others?

Completion of the literature review enables the researcher to revisit the original research idea and define the exact focus of the research problem. The literature review should put the research problem into context. A good literature review contains an up-to-date resumé of the literature and a balanced review of differing viewpoints or findings. Reviewing the literature is not simply a case of identifying previous research; it involves critical appraisal of the merits of the research. In writing up the results of a literature search the researcher should present a logical coherent case for pursuing the study.

Detailed information on how to search and review the literature can be found in the Trent Focus research volume *Developing Research in Primary Care*, Chapter 2 'Carrying out a literature review'.

Methodology

Once the researcher has decided on the focus of the project, the next stage is to develop a plan of investigation. In developing the plan the researcher takes into consideration such things as:

- what am I trying to find out?
- what sort of information do I need?
- what is the best way to collect the information?
- where can I get the information from?
- how many people will I need to ask?
- how will I analyse and make sense of the information I collect?

The term 'methodology' refers to all these matters regarding the structure and design of the research study. It deals with such issues as:

- the type of information required
- the research design
- the method of collecting data
- the source of information – this is known as the 'sample'.

Type of information

This depends on the original research idea. If the researcher wants to collect measurable information about a topic this is referred to as 'quantitative research'. It looks at:

- how big the problem is
- how many people are affected by it
- how often something occurs
- is one thing more or less important than another?
- do some things occur more often than others?

The specific elements that the researcher tries to measure are called 'variables'. The outcomes that the researcher is trying to establish are variables – for example, degree of pain, recovery time, levels of improvement, satisfaction. Variables are also the features that may have an effect on the outcomes, for example a patient's age, weight or nutritional state.

Some situations cannot be easily broken down into a set of variables. The best example is human behaviour: why people act the way they do or how they feel in certain circumstances. If the researcher is trying to understand something in more detail or to describe a situation so that people can understand it better, this is often better achieved through qualitative research. In qualitative research, attention is focused on answering questions such as:

- why?
- in what way?
- what are the implications?

rather than, how many? how often? how much?, as occurs in quantitative research. Further features of quantitative and qualitative research are listed in Box 1.2.

Box 1.2   Features of quantitative and qualitative research

Quantitative

- the emphasis is on collecting measurable information
- data can be analysed statistically
- data can be quickly collected so large samples can be used
- data can be collected from a distance so it can be collected from widely dispersed members of the population
- data collection tools are highly structured and are time-consuming to develop
- once the tool is developed, data collection is relatively quick and cheap to collect and analyse
- the main forms of data collection are: questionnaire surveys, highly structured observation schedules and analysis of records

Qualitative

- information can only be loosely measured: the main issues can be identified but not specifically measured
- data cannot be statistically analysed
- data collection is more time-consuming so uses smaller samples
- data are usually collected face to face, so collecting data from a widely dispersed sample is time-consuming and expensive – local samples tend to used
- data collection tools are more loosely structured
- data collection and data analysis are time-consuming and comparatively expensive
- the main forms of data collection are individual interviews, focus groups and less-structured observation

---

The research design

After deciding on the type of data required, qualitative or quantitative, the next methodological decision to be taken is on the type of research that will best address the research problem. There are many different types of research design. The choice of design depends on the research problem. Research can be carried out using experiments, correlation studies, surveys, case studies, action research, ethnography, grounded theory, and phenomenology.

Experimental designs

Experiments are controlled investigations that try to establish cause and effect between two or more variables with the purpose of predicting outcomes – for example, whether one type of medication is more effective than another in treating a particular illness. There are several different kinds of experimental design, but the classic experimental design involves two groups, an intervention group and a control group. Information relevant to the research problem is collected on the subjects (people) in both groups. Then one group, the intervention group, receives some kind of special or different treatment (the intervention) while the control group receives no treatment or the usual treatment. Information is then collected from both groups and analysed to see whether the outcomes of the two groups are different or the same. Experiments are carried out by collecting quantitative data that are subjected to statistical tests, which assess the probability that the variables are linked in a cause-and-effect relationship. Further information is contained in Chapter 2 *Experimental designs*.

Correlation studies

Like experimental designs, correlation studies also investigate the likelihood of a relationship between two variables but they are interested in identifying associations rather than cause and effect. For example, is there a relationship between social group and the number of GP consultations? A correlation study might find that patients from a certain social group are more likely than patients from other social groups to visit the GP for certain kinds of health problems. A correlation study does not prove that the patient is going to the GP because s/he is from a particular social group. The findings are limited to demonstrating that there is an association. That is, that patients from that group are more likely to consult the GP. Correlation studies collect quantitative data, which are subjected to statistical tests that calculate the strength of the link – the correlation.

Surveys

A survey involves asking individuals questions about their opinions, beliefs, attitudes or behaviours with regard to a given topic. Individuals are selected to take part in a survey because they share certain characteristics and form some kind of population. They may be questioned by asking them to complete a questionnaire, by face-to-face interview or by telephone interview. Examples of surveys in primary healthcare include investigations of patient satisfaction and lifestyle studies. Small-scale surveys involving a small number of participants may collect either qualitative or quantitative information, but larger scale studies involving hundreds or even thousands of people would collect quantitative data. The survey is one of the most frequently used research designs and is popular with first-time researchers. Most people have been asked to take part in a survey at some time. More information on surveys can be found in Chapter 4 *Surveys and questionnaires*.

Case studies

Case studies are in-depth investigations of a single or small number of units. The unit may be individual people, patients, groups or organisations. One of the most common uses of the case-study method is evaluation of a service – for example, a drop-in facility, providing advice and support for teenagers. Another example would be an examination of team building in one or a small number of primary healthcare teams. Case studies involve the collection of qualitative or quantitative information, or a combination of both.

Action research

Action research is used to investigate the effects of interventions in real-life situations that involve practitioners. It is often used when practitioners want to change their way of working, when introducing a new service, or to increase their efficiency or effectiveness. It is a problem-solving approach that involves the team in a process of reflecting on their situation, identifying problems and possible responses, implementing the change and evaluating the effects. Action research is often described as cyclical in nature because the team may go through the process of reflection–identification–intervention–evaluation several times. An example of action research might be the introduction of a nurse-led primary healthcare service. Like case studies, the researcher often collects a combination of qualitative and quantitative data.

Ethnography

Ethnography is a form of qualitative research. It is used to investigate cultures and population subgroups and seeks to explore, describe and explain cultural behaviour – for example understanding of mental illness within a particular Asian subgroup. In primary healthcare, ethnography helps healthcare professionals to develop cultural awareness and adapt existing services to develop new approaches to meet patients' needs. As a form of qualitative research, ethnography requires the collection of in-depth information through face-to-face contact with individuals over a period of time. Analysis of data concentrates on understanding and describing the situation from the perspective of the culture or subgroup under study.

Phenomenology

Phenomenology literally means the study of phenomena. It is a way of describing elements that are part of the world in which we live: events, situations, experiences or concepts. Phenomenological research investigates individuals' lived experience of events.

An introduction to research methodology

It asks questions like: 'what does it mean to the individual to be involved in this situation, what effect does it have on that individual's life, their feelings and their behaviour?' One example of phenomenological research would be an investigation into the experience of caring for someone with senile dementia. The study would consider the meaning of caring in that context, the components of caring and the impact – negative and positive – it has on carers' lives.

Grounded theory

This is a form of research that goes beyond collecting and analysing data to add to the existing body of knowledge. In grounded theory, the emphasis is on developing new knowledge and new theories about the topic being investigated.

Ethnography, phenomenology and grounded theory are all research designs based on the collection of qualitative data. Further information can be found in Chapter 3 *Qualitative research*.

Exercise 2

Listed below are examples of proposed research projects to be undertaken in primary healthcare settings. Consider each one and suggest the most appropriate research design.

1. What are patients' views of the range of services provided by the local health centre?
2. What factors are likely to influence the uptake of screening services among women aged 16–50 years?
3. The use of homeopathic treatments by the Chinese population in one city in England.
4. How successfully can eating disorders be treated by GPs? A study of three teenage girls.
5. What is the most effective and efficient method of providing counselling to treat depression in primary care: counselling by GPs or counselling by community psychiatric nurses (CPNs)?
6. How to decrease interruptions during practice nurse consultations in one general practice.

Methods of collecting data

Having decided on how to design the research study, the next methodological decision is how to collect information. The most commonly used methods of collecting information are interviews, questionnaires and observation.

Interviews

Interviews are usually held on a one-to-one basis, but some studies may use group interviews or focus groups. Interviews can be highly structured, semi-structured or unstructured. The degree of structure affects the flexibility of the interview. Guidance on using interviews to collect data can be found in Chapter 5 *Using interviews in a research project*.

Questionnaires

Questionnaires comprise a written set of questions that are answered by all respondents in a study. Several different types of questions can be used. Closed questions seek a limited response. If a range of responses can be predicted in advance – for example, eye colour – the respondent may be provided with a pre-set list of answers to choose from. At the other end of the scale, open questions allow the respondent to answer freely in their own words and are used when a more extensive response is being sought, for example an explanation. Questionnaires are often used to assess attitudes, and respondents may be asked to choose a point on a scale, either semantic or numeric, to indicate how they perceive or feel about a situation. Guidance on using questionnaires to collect data can be found in Chapter 4 *Surveys and questionnaires*.

Observation

Observation is a technique for collecting data through visual observation of events. It requires the nature of the data to be observable. Like the other two methods of collecting data, observation schedules can be highly structured or relatively unstructured, depending on the type of information required and the nature of the observed event. Guidance on using observation to collect data can be found in Chapter 6 *Data collection by observation*.

The method of data collection chosen for a study should be appropriate for the type of information required. Whether the required information is quantitative or qualitative in nature is the major consideration. It would be time wasting to use unstructured interviews for essentially quantitative studies where information could be more efficiently collected through structured interviews or questionnaires. Conversely, self-completed questionnaires are generally unsuited to qualitative research: even when there is space for comments or for respondents to express ideas, the space is limited and requires respondents to have skills in articulation and literacy.

The advantages and disadvantages of the different methods of collecting data are summarised in Boxes 1.3, 1.4 and 1.5.

It is not always necessary to design a new data collection tool for a research project. During the literature search the researcher may discover a questionnaire that suits the intended purpose. It is acceptable to use data-collection tools that have been developed by previous researchers. It may even be preferable since the tool is more likely to have been subjected to tests for reliability and validity.

An introduction to research methodology

Box 1.3   Advantages and disadvantages of the interview

Advantages

1. No items are overlooked.
2. Questions and answers can be clarified by both interviewer and interviewee.
3. Researcher can achieve depth of response.
4. Can be used to probe sensitive or difficult areas.
5. Good response rates.
6. Interviewees don't need to be able to read or write to participate.
7. Interviewees' responses are not influenced by reading ahead (can happen with questionnaires).
8. Responses are enriched by observing non-verbal cues and paralinguistics.
9. Can be used as an exploratory stage in a larger study.

Disadvantages

1. Takes time to arrange.
2. Time-consuming for researcher as takes longer to collect data.
3. Travelling can be costly.
4. Interview skills are needed.
5. Risk of interviewer bias.
6. Data analysis can be time-consuming.

Box 1.4   Advantages and disadvantages of the questionnaire

Advantages

1. Relatively simple method of collecting data. Novice researchers can design simple questionnaires.
2. Rapid and efficient method of gathering data.
3. Can collect data from a widely scattered sample.
4. Can collect data from a large sample.
5. Relatively inexpensive.
6. Respondents can remain anonymous.
7. One of easiest tools to test for reliability and validity.
8. Respondent has time to consider each question.
9. Analysis of data can be done quickly.
10. Can be used to collect data on a wide range of topics/attributes.

Disadvantages

1. Cannot probe a topic in-depth without being lengthy.
2. Respondent can omit items without explanation, therefore data incomplete.
3. Selection of forced choice items may be insufficient to reflect respondent's choice.
4. Amount of information limited by respondent's interest and attention.
5. Questionnaires can go astray.
6. Production and distribution can become expensive.
7. Sample is limited to those with literacy skills.
8. Most people express themselves better through the spoken word.
9. No opportunity for researcher to interact with respondents.
10. If respondents are anonymous they cannot be followed up.

> **Box 1.5 Advantages and disadvantages of observation**
>
> **Advantages**
>
> 1. Best way of recording human behaviour.
> 2. Observations recorded as they occur, eliminating biased recall.
> 3. Allows researcher to view a situation in total and in context.
> 4. Observation schedules can be simple to design and use.
> 5. Observers may need little training.
> 6. Open to the use of recording devices.
>
> **Disadvantages**
>
> 1. Time and duration of an event may not be predictable; involves watching and waiting.
> 2. Presence of observer adds a new dimension to the situation.
> 3. Presence of observer can affect people's behaviour.
> 4. Observations may be subject to observer bias.
> 5. Observers may find themselves drawn into the situation.
> 6. Events may occur so rapidly it is not possible to record everything.
> 7. Little control over number of times an event will occur.
> 8. Those not wishing to be involved may object to the presence of the observer.

Sampling

In any research the researcher has to identify the population under study. If a GP wants to carry out research about patients he needs to decide if this means any type of patient or if he is interested in a particular section of the practice population. Furthermore, if he eventually decides that the research is actually about, for example, 'older people', the minimum age or alternative criteria should be identified. If the target population is large it may not be feasible to include everyone in the research so a sample has to be selected. There are different ways of sampling and the most common ways are summarised below. There are reasons to use different approaches to sampling and each approach has strengths and weaknesses.

Random sampling

This is a method that gives every member of the population a calculable chance (often equal) of being selected. It is frequently described as the method of sampling least likely to produce a bias, but sampling errors can occur by chance which can unintentionally produce bias.

Stratified sampling

This is used when the population contains subgroups and it is necessary to ensure that representatives of all groups are included, e.g. patients in different age bands, nurses employed on different professional grades, healthcare staff from a range of professions. Randomisation within each subgroup can be applied.

Systematic sampling

This involves taking the *nth* name on a list, such as every third person or every tenth. Unless the list is arranged randomly, the sample will not be random. This approach may eliminate certain members of the population who may have a perspective which is useful to the study but go unnoticed, e.g. taking the first named member of the household from an electoral roll will almost certainly eliminate the younger members of the population.

Cluster sampling

This is used when the population is diversely spread over a geographical area, where for various reasons it is preferable to include groups of subjects from several sites rather than randomly selecting the whole sample from the whole population. An example of this would be: to investigate the grades of community nurses employed nationally the sample could select a sample of community nurses in one NHS trust in each of the health regions.

Convenience sampling

Also called incidental sampling, this method utilises readily available subjects and is often used in qualitative projects and hypothesis generating. The sample may not be representative of the population as a whole and the results may not be generalisable, e.g. patients selected from one geographical area such as an electoral ward may have particularly high or low levels of deprivation.

Sequential sampling

The size of the sample is not pre-set. The researcher collects data from each subject in turn until he is satisfied that there is no new information for collection – the topic is saturated. It is used mostly in qualitative research, e.g. in setting up a new service, potential users are asked what they would want until no new ideas emerge.

Purposive sampling

Subjects are selected because they have certain characteristics, e.g. key stakeholders in an organisation.

Exercise 3

What type of sample has been used in the four studies outlined below?

1. Practice nurses in four general practices decide to investigate the incidence and causation of interruptions during consultations. They survey all interruptions in their own practices over a four-week period.
2. The Health Education Authority wants to know what kind of Well Man clinics are provided in general practice. It writes to a quarter of the practice managers in every health authority to ask for information.
3. The Royal College of Nursing wants to know what arrangements are in place for clinical supervision among community psychiatric nurses. It asks every regional office to select one health trust and to send questionnaires to all team leaders in the trust.
4. A community dietician wants to know what nutritional advice is needed by newly diagnosed cancer patients. She decides to interview all new referrals until she stops getting new information.

Access and ethical issues

In trying to access the sample the researcher has to consider how this can practically be achieved and whose permission must be sought. Access to patients normally requires permission from the responsible medical officer or the NHS trust. Access to staff requires permission from their manager. By seeking permission to contact the sample group the researcher is also more likely to secure practical help and advice to access subjects.

The researcher must also consider any ethical implications of the research. At the very least this involves issues of confidentiality and anonymity, but there may be other factors to consider which, unless resolved, could potentially have negative implications for the subjects directly or indirectly. For example, research which tests the effectiveness of new treatment approaches may eventually show that the new treatment is better than the old, but in order to find out, it may be necessary to withhold the established treatment from a sample group of patients. Any risks associated with this should be carefully assessed.

The researcher should seek advice and if necessary formal permission to undertake the study from the local research ethics committee. Advice on identifying ethical issues for consideration and how to apply for ethical approval can be found in the Trent Focus volume *Developing Research in Primary Care*, Chapter 3 'Ethical considerations in research'.

The pilot study

Once the researcher is ready to undertake the study s/he should carry out a small pilot study to check that the methodology has been thought through correctly. The pilot is the study in miniature and gives the researcher an opportunity to identify any problems and to modify the research method before embarking on the main study.

The pilot study enables the researcher to check the following:

- the accessibility of the sample group
- the likely response rate
- whether or not the data-collection tool provides the depth, range and quality of information required.

If problems are detected at the pilot study stage the researcher has the opportunity to make revisions before undertaking the main study. This increases the likelihood that the data collected in the main study will be usable.

Data collection

Once the methodology has been thought through and the method of data collection has been piloted, the researcher reaches the stage of conducting the interviews, sending out the questionnaires or recording observations. For many researchers, this is the most exciting or enjoyable part of the research process. After what can sometimes be weeks or months of planning – developing the research idea, reviewing the literature, designing the research approach – the researcher starts to investigate the topic through the collection of original data.

Data analysis

This is the next stage of the research process, when the researcher reviews the data collected and systematically analyses the responses of subjects. Up to this point every participant's responses form a separate record. Combining all these separate records into one and providing an overview produces the results of a research study.

Data are described, summarised and, if quantitative in nature, statistically analysed in order to produce the results of the study. The techniques employed in data analysis are dependent on the type of information collected, the research design and the design of the data-collection tool. As we have already seen, qualitative and quantitative data are very different in content and require very different approaches.

Qualitative data is analysed by reading respondents' comments (questionnaires and interview transcripts), or by listening to their comments (tape-recorded interviews) or by reviewing their behaviour (observation). The range of responses is described and examples of behaviour or narrative are used to illustrate both the typicality and diversity of responses. More detailed information on the analysis of qualitative data can be found in Chapter 3 *Qualitative research*.

Quantitative data are analysed by counting the frequency with which certain features occur among participants' responses. The summarised data can then be subjected to a variety of statistical measures to identify patterns or trends (descriptive statistics) and to assess what inferences can be made from the data about the general population (inferential statistics). (More information about this can be found in the Trent Focus volume *Statistical Analysis in Primary Care*, Chapter 1 'An introduction to using statistics'.) If the research project is a small-scale study with data collection from a small sample and the researcher does not want to carry out sophisticated statistical analysis, it should be possible to analyse the data by hand. If not, then it is advisable to use computerised software packages. They require the data to be inputted manually, although the computer does the hard work of calculating and comparing the results. An introduction to two of the most widely used statistical packages is in the Trent Focus volume *Statistical Analysis in Primary Care*, Chapters 3 and 4 'An introduction to using SPSS' and 'An introduction to using Epi Info'.

Drawing conclusions

When the data have been analysed and a full set of results has been produced, the researcher reviews the results and considers them in the context of previous knowledge. This final stage of the research process contains three key elements:

- discussing the findings
- identifying the limitations of the study
- making recommendations for further research and for practice.

The results are considered in light of the original research problem. If this was stated as an aim, the researcher discusses the extent to which the aim was achieved. If the research problem was stated as a question, the researcher considers whether the research study has provided an answer. If a hypothesis was used, the researcher has to decide whether it can be accepted or rejected according to the results.

Considering the overall strengths and weaknesses of the study design and the results identifies the limitations of the research project. For example, the size or selection of the sample may limit the generalisability of the results, or the depth and breadth of data may limit the conclusions that can be drawn. It is important that the limitations of a study are always recognised, as readers should take them into consideration when deciding whether or not to act on the results of the study.

Finally, consideration is given to how the results could be applied to practice. At the beginning of this chapter it was stated that research is intended to add to the body of knowledge, but if the limitations are extensive, the research will have limited value. Caution should therefore be exercised in recommending changes to current practice or making unrealistic claims about the extent to which knowledge can be informed by the findings. In this case it is more appropriate for the researcher to identify the need for further research and to make recommendations about the direction that the research could take.

Summary

This chapter has provided a brief overview of the research process. We have looked at the sequence of steps taken by researchers as they plan a research project, undertake the project and make sense of the findings. The information on methodology has shown that there are different types of research and that the choice of method depends on the research problem, the type of information needed and practical matters such as the time and resources available to carry out the research.

Depending on previous knowledge, the chapter may have acted as an introduction or as a reminder of the main elements of the research process. It is hoped that readers will feel encouraged to look at the other titles in the Trent Focus series, although the selection of chapters will depend on where further interests lie: in using, doing, or implementing research.

Exercise 4

In this exercise you have the opportunity to revisit the research process in total and to assess how much you have remembered. Listed below are ten questions, each one requires a short answer. Try to answer all the questions before checking your answers at the end of the chapter. If you didn't understand some of the questions or answered incorrectly, you are advised to reread the appropriate section.

1. What are the three ways of stating the purpose of the research, i.e. the research problem?
2. Why is it important to undertake a review of the literature before planning a research project?
3. You want to know more about the demographic details of your client group, how often they seek advice on health-related issues and how often they suffer from a range of 'minor' health issues. What research design could you use?
4. Name one type of qualitative research design.
5. Name one type of quantitative research design.
6. List the three main methods of collecting information.
7. If you wanted to collect quantitative data from 1000 people spread over a wide geographical area, what method of data collection would you be most likely to use?
8. What is the difference between random sampling and convenience sampling?
9. Why is it important to conduct a pilot study?
10. When you read the conclusions of a research study, what three key elements would you hope to find?

Answers to exercises

Exercise 1

aim: The aim of the research is to investigate patient satisfaction with the appointments system.
question: Are patients satisfied with the appointments system?
hypothesis: There is a link between levels of patient satisfaction and the operation of the appointments system.

Exercise 2

1. Survey.
2. Correlation study.
3. Ethnography.
4. Case study.
5. Experimental design.
6. Action research.

Exercise 3

1. Convenience sample.
2. Random sample.
3. Cluster sample.
4. Sequential sample.

Exercise 4

1. Research problems can be stated as aims, questions or hypotheses.
2. The literature review provides information about: what is currently known about the topic, what aspects of the topic lack sufficient information, previous research, recommendations for further research made previously but not acted upon, methods used by previous researchers to investigate the topic.
3. The survey.
4. Phenomenology, ethnography and grounded theory are all qualitative research designs. However, action research, case studies and surveys can also be used qualitatively.
5. Experimental designs and correlation studies are quantitative research designs. Large-scale surveys usually collect quantitative data and case studies may also be quantitative in orientation.

6. Interviews, questionnaires and observation.
7. The questionnaire.
8. In a randomly selected sample everyone in the defined population has an equal chance of being selected. A random sample is technically free of bias and should be representative of the population. A convenience sample utilises readily available subjects and they may not be sufficiently representative of the population.
9. The pilot study enables the researcher to check:
   - the accessibility of the sample group
   - the likely response rate
   - whether or not the data-collection tool provides the depth, range and quality of information required.

   If problems are detected at the pilot study stage, the researcher has the opportunity to make revisions before undertaking the main study. This increases the likelihood that the data collected in the main study will be usable.
10. A discussion of the findings in relation to the original research problem; the limitations of the study; recommendations for practice and/or further research.

CHAPTER TWO

Experimental designs

Heather Wharrad

Introduction

The aim of this chapter is to provide an overview of the principles underlying experimental research design to allow the reader to be able to read research literature and evaluate research proposals critically.

This includes the following objectives:

- to introduce the reader to experimental method as it relates to primary healthcare
- to describe different experimental designs and give examples of when they may be used
- to determine when the experimental approach is an appropriate research method for a particular research question
- to identify strengths and weaknesses of the experimental method.

Identifying the problem

The word 'experimenting' is used in our everyday language to describe our actions when we are testing or trying out something new, for example 'I am experimenting with this new recipe' or 'they are experimenting with a different team'. In such situations the experimentation is performed, albeit unwittingly, in a fairly *ad hoc* or 'uncontrolled' manner. In experimental research, however, the design and progress of an experiment is carefully controlled by the researcher.

Any research problem is inevitably multifactorial in nature. Let us consider an example. A health worker might wish to investigate the development of pressure sores in patients. Many factors, in this context known as *variables*, might influence the development of pressure sores, such as:

- psychological condition
- age
- sex

- mobility
- mattress
- nursing practice
- nutrition
- medical/surgical intervention
- number of sores
- grade of sores
- size of sores.

Some of the variables relate to the physical characteristics or condition of the patient, others relate to the medical or nursing interventions which the patient has experienced. Descriptions of the pressure sores themselves are also variables, so the number of sores, the size of sores and the grade of sore are all variables.

Dependent and independent variables

In experimental research, the researcher manipulates one or more of the variables – these are termed the *independent variables* – and monitors how subjects react by measuring a response in one or more outcome measures or *dependent variables*. In the simplest experimental design, a researcher might manipulate just one independent variable and measure a change in one dependent variable, so in our list above, a health worker might investigate the relationship between mobility (the independent variable) and the grade of pressure sore which develops in a patient (dependent variable). If a researcher wanted to investigate the effect of posture on pulse rate, s/he might measure pulse rate in a group of subjects who were sitting, then repeat the measurement with the subjects standing. Here the posture adopted is the independent variable as this is the variable being changed by the experimenter. The dependent variable is pulse rate – this is the variable being measured during the experiment. The change in the independent variable is planned by the researcher before the experiment is carried out, whereas how the dependent variable will change is not known until the experiment has been performed – it is 'dependent' on the change in the independent variable.

Exercise 1

Hofman A, Geelkerken R H, Wille J, Hamming J J, Breslau P J (1994) Pressure sores and pressure-decreasing mattresses: controlled clinical trial. *Lancet.* **343**: 568–71.

Summary
Pressure sores are a problem, especially in elderly patients. Our study was designed to determine the effectiveness in pressure-sore prevention of a new interface pressure-decreasing mattress.

Experimental designs

In a prospective randomised controlled trial we tested the Comfortex DeCube mattress (Comfortex, Winona USA) against our standard mattress in 44 patients with femoral-neck fracture and concomitant high pressure-sore risk score. In addition both groups were treated according to the Dutch consensus protocol for the prevention of pressure sores. On admission, and one and two weeks after admission, pressure sores were graded. The two groups were similar in patient characteristics and pressure-sore risk factors. At one week, 25% of the patients nursed on the DeCube mattress and 64% of the patients nursed on the standard mattress had clinically relevant pressure sores (grade 2 or more). At two weeks the figures were 24% and 68% respectively. The maximum score over the several body regions of the pressure-sore grading, measured on a 5-point scale, was significantly different in favour of the DeCube mattress at one week ($p=0.0043$) and two weeks ($p=0.0067$) post-operatively.

We show that the occurrence of pressure sores and their severity can be significantly reduced when patients at risk are nursed on an interface pressure-decreasing mattress.

1. What is the dependent variable in this experiment?
2. What is the independent variable?

As we shall see later in this chapter, more complex experimental designs allow the investigation of the relationships between a number of independent and dependent variables within one experiment. One word of warning, though, a common mistake made by inexperienced (and sometimes more experienced!) researchers is to try to address too many research questions in one experiment. This not only leads to difficulties when analysing and interpreting the data, but also can be time-consuming for researchers and subjects alike.

The results of a well-designed experiment, along with appropriate statistical analyses (see the Trent Focus research volume *Statistical Analysis in Primary Care*), allow the experimenter to make inferences about possible associations between the independent and dependent variables. The next section will introduce the basic principles behind experimental designs.

Basic principles of experimental design

Developing research questions and formulating hypotheses

Research questions develop from the identification of a 'problem' or 'issue' derived from our own professional experiences within the healthcare setting and from studying relevant literature on the subject. From these questions we formulate *hypotheses* to test. A *hypothesis* is a testable proposition about the outcome of an experiment, or an 'educated guess' based on your knowledge and experience about how the independent variable will affect the dependent variable. Every experiment tests at least one hypothesis, more often several hypotheses, in each case predicting the relationship between variables.

Exercise 2

The hypothesis is often not overtly stated in published research papers. Can you identify the statement in the extract in Exercise 1 that indicates the research question?

Null hypothesis

Experimental research relies on statistical analysis to determine whether the change in the independent variable is related to the change in the dependent variable. Statistical analysis is the subject of the Trent Focus research volume *Statistical Analysis in Primary Care*. However, it is worth introducing at this point the term *null hypothesis*, a statement of no difference or no relationship between the variables and a fundamental concept on which all statistical tests are based.

Examples of null hypotheses
1. There is no difference in pulse rate in the sitting and standing positions.
2. Mobility has no effect on grade of pressure sore.
3. Drug x has no effect on diastolic blood pressure.

Exercise 3

Try altering the statement below into a null hypothesis – it is the one posed in the extract in Exercise 1.

> 'Our study was designed to determine the effectiveness in pressure-sore prevention of a new interface pressure-decreasing mattress.'

To reiterate the important point made in the introduction, the more complex the pattern of interaction of variables, the less likely it is an experiment can be designed. It is worth remembering that when asking broad questions about subjects' opinions, a *qualitative* approach might be considered as a more appropriate research method.

Selection and manipulation of variables

One essential component of the experimental design is the evaluation of manipulated change, the assumption is made that the dependent variable will not vary unless the independent variable changes. The independent variable is often termed the *intervention*.

Experimental designs

The choice of independent and dependent variables should be carefully considered. This section summarises the factors to take into account when selecting the dependent and independent variables for your experiment.

Reliability

A measurement tool is said to be reliable if it can be consistently used by other researchers to obtain reproducible results when applied in an identical (as far as is possible) setting. If the dependent variable was something fairly simple, like height or weight, the choice of measurement instrument is not a problem. However, even with these simple instruments, it is important to further standardise the measurement by defining standard conditions to be followed when making the measurement, such as removing shoes and checking that the scales are zeroed before each measurement. The omission of even simple instructions such as these can lead to unreliable results, particularly if different researchers are making the measurements. Consider another fairly simple measurement, estimation of arterial blood pressure using a sphygmomanometer; there are four main sources of variation and error in the technique leading to unreliability in this measurement: the observer, the patient, the technique and the equipment. These have been published in more detail in a paper by O'Brian and Davison (1994). Factors that enhance the accuracy of arterial blood pressure measurement and recording are listed in Table 2.1.

Table 2.1 Factors to consider when standardising the technique for blood pressure measurement that enhance the accuracy of the recording (adapted from O'Brian and Davison 1994)

Patient	Sitting or lying for at least 3 minutes
	No clothing on arm
	Arm supported level with heart
	Psychologically calm
	No recent smoking or alcohol consumption
Equipment	Matching cuff dimensions to patient's arm circumference
	Sphygmomanometer calibrated 6-monthly
	Sphygmomanometer and stethoscope regularly maintained
Observer	Agreement about phase IV and V Korotkoff sounds for diastolic pressure
	Reading to the nearest 2 mmHg, i.e. no rounding to the nearest 5 or 10 mmHg
	Patient's arm adequately supported
	Cuff fitted firmly
	Centre of bladder cuff over brachial artery

These considerations are important for health workers in practice as well as for researchers. If there are variations in the way blood pressure is recorded by different researchers, then a true change in blood pressure due to an intervention might be missed. An erroneous reading which is consistently made by an observer, such as always rounding up the reading to the nearest 5 mmHg instead of reading to the nearest 2 mmHg, is called a *systematic error*.

It is also important that the intervention (the independent variable) is applied in exactly the same way to all the subjects throughout the experiment. In the same way that the measurement of the dependent variable is *standardised*, so should the application of the independent variable. This is achieved by verifying techniques and by using a standard protocol. A pilot study will verify whether the protocol is workable. Pilot studies are described later in this chapter.

Exercise 4

Which other errors in blood-pressure measurement might be considered to be systematic errors?

Validity

Measurement tools also need to be valid. A valid test or tool is one which measures what it purports to measure. There is a good example which is commonly used to explain the concept of validity (Clegg 1994). You can use a tape-measure to determine head size and record it in centimetres and thus have a perfectly reliable measurement which would be reproducible if other people repeated the same measurement. It is also a valid measurement of head size. However, if you were to use it as a measure of intelligence, then the measurement is still reliable but it is certainly not valid!

Intelligence is an example of many important dimensions of human subjects that are so complex and multivariate that it is impossible to gain universal agreement about how it can be measured validly and reliably.

Exercise 5

Before reading on, spend a minute or two thinking about other aspects of human behaviour or experiences that might come under this category.

Some of the aspects of human behaviour you might have come up with are:

- pain
- stress or anxiety
- healthcare
- attitudes
- personality.

Some workers have used physiological or biochemical indices to measure changes in stress or pain. For example Boore *et al.* (1978) measured levels of corticosteroids excreted as her dependent variable for determining stress levels. Some researchers argue that this

Experimental designs

Box 2.1		
Dependent variable	**Measurement tool**	**Experimental study using tool**
pain	McGill pain questionnaire (MPQ)	Pain on a surgical ward Melzack et al. (1987)
anxiety	Spielberger STAI-X1	Who's afraid of informed consent? Kerrigan et al. (1993)

reductionist approach in order to obtain objectivity is inappropriate for human subjects. Many 'tools' in the form of questionnaires are now available for assessing these complex emotions in a more holistic way (see examples in Box 2.1). These types of tools require consideration of what is termed *content validity*. This means does the instrument (questionnaire) include all the relevant questions related to the hypothesis? In other words, will this tool give valid results for the research question being investigated?

Where a recognised reliable or valid measurement tool for assessing the dependent variable does not exist, researchers must develop one themselves, ensuring to check it for reliability and validity.

Potency

It is important to ensure that the intervention is of sufficient potency to produce a measurable change in the dependent variable, otherwise we assume wrongly that an intervention has no effect (in statistics this is termed a Type II error). The simplest example of this is giving a drug in too low a dose. In drug trials early experiments take the form of a dose-response curve to find out which dose is effective.

Example

In a trial of the effect of advice to stop smoking on middle-aged men, the intervention was a series of information-giving interviews. The experimenters felt that to change an entrenched behaviour such as smoking habits by providing information via a pamphlet or booklet, rather than using interviews, was unlikely to be a potent enough intervention (Rose et al. 1978).

Pilot study

The procedures and protocol of an experiment are normally tested on a small number of people prior to the main study. A pilot study is a trial run. It allows researchers to check whether equipment is functioning properly or whether respondents understand the phrasing of questions in a questionnaire. It is rare, however well planned, for a few unforeseen problems not to arise in the course of an experiment. The subjects who take part in the pilot study should be from the same general population as the subjects selected for the main study.

Example
Roe B H (1990) Study of the effects of education on patients' knowledge and acceptance of in-dwelling urethral catheters. *J. Adv. Nursing.* **15**: 223–31.

> 'The information booklet, written on the basis of a literature review, was tested at a pre-pilot stage by lay people (non-catheter users) who were asked to check its readability and sense. Amendments were made and it was then formally tested in the pilot study.'

Control groups

Consideration of the independent variables leads neatly on to the discussion of the term *control*. If the aim of the experimental method is to determine the relationship between the independent and dependent variables, it is obviously important to ensure that all the other known possible influences are held constant. Thinking back to the classic experiments we did at school in plant biology, it was fairly easy to keep constant factors other than those we were investigating so when looking at the effect of light on leaf colour we could ensure that temperature, amounts of water etc. were identical for all plants in the experiment; that is we control for as many of these unwanted factors as possible. The only variable manipulated would be the independent variable – light. These unwanted factors are called *extraneous variables*. When they are likely to affect the dependent variable they are known as *confounding variables*.

In human research, controlling other variables is more problematic than in botany or the physical sciences! The complexities of human behaviour mean that not only is it difficult to eliminate confounding variables, but it is often impossible to identify all of them in the first place!

One way of accounting for any influence of confounding variables on the dependent variables is by means of a *control group*. Subjects in the control group do not receive the intervention or treatment and they therefore act as a *baseline* against which the effects of the intervention can be measured. Without a control group it is difficult for researchers

Experimental designs

to be sure that the observed change in the dependent variable was solely due to the independent variable or due to other influences (confounding variables).

In recent years the nature of the control group has changed. Rather than receiving no treatment, control groups may receive a standard or minimal treatment against which the effect of a new treatment can be compared. This change has arisen due to the raised awareness of ethical responsibility. It is not ethical to withdraw or withhold a beneficial treatment in a group of control subjects simply to satisfy the conditions of experimental research.

Exercise 6

The first extract below summarises a study describing the effect of mattress type on the development of pressure sores. List the confounding variables that might have influenced the dependent variables in this study – you may find the list on pages 23–24 helpful!

1. Kerrigan D D *et al.* (1993) Who's afraid of informed consent? *BMJ*. **306**: 298–300.
   Objective – To test the assumption that patients will become unduly anxious if they are given detailed information about the risks of surgery in an attempt to gain fully informed consent.
   Design – Pre-operative anxiety assessed before and after patients were randomly allocated an information sheet containing either simple or detailed descriptions of possible post-operative complications.
   Setting – Four surgical wards at two Sheffield hospitals.
   Subjects – 96 men undergoing elective inguinal hernia repair under general anaesthetic.
   Main outcome measure – Change in anxiety level observed after receiving information about potential complications.
   Results – Detailed information did not increase patient anxiety (mean Spielberger score at baseline 33.7 (95% confidence interval 31.3 to 36.2), after information 34.8 (32.1 to 37.5); p=0.20, paired t-test). A simple explanation of the facts provided a statistically significant degree of reassurance (mean score at baseline 34.6 (31.5 to 37.6), after information 32.3 (29.8 to 34.9); p=0.012), although this small effect is likely to be clinically important only in those whose baseline anxiety was high (r=0.27, p=0.05).
   Conclusions – In men undergoing elective inguinal hernia repair a very detailed account of what might go wrong does not increase patient anxiety significantly and has the advantage of allowing patients a fully informed choice before they consent to surgery, thus reducing the potential for subsequent litigation.
2. Sleep J *et al.* (1984) West Berkshire perineal management trial. *BMJ*. **289**: 587–90.
   One thousand women were allocated at random to one of two perineal management policies, both intended to minimise trauma during spontaneous vaginal delivery. In one the aim was to restrict episiotomy to fetal indications; in the other the operation was to be used more liberally to prevent perineal tears. The resultant episiotomy rates were 10% and 51% respectively. An intact perineum was more

common among those allocated to the restrictive policy. This group experienced more perineal and labial tears, however, and included four of the five cases of severe trauma. There were no significant differences between the two groups either in neonatal state or in maternal pain and urinary symptoms ten days and three months post-partum. Women allocated to the restrictive policy were more likely to have resumed sexual intercourse within a month of delivery.

These findings provide little support either for liberal use of episiotomy or for claims that reduced use of the operation decreased post-partum morbidity.

Exercise 7

From the extract in Exercise 1, and the two extracts above, complete Box 2.2, indicating what the 'control' treatment is in each study.

Box 2.2

Study	Authors	Description of control group
Extract 1: Pressure sores and pressure-decreasing mattresses controlled clinical trial	Hofman A et al. (1994) Lancet. **343**: 568–71	
Extract 2: Who's afraid of informed consent?	Kerrigan D D et al. (1993) BMJ. **306**: 298–300	
Extract 3: West Berkshire perineal management trial	Sleep J et al. (1984) BMJ. **289**: 587–90	

The placebo

The introduction of placebo-controlled drug trials in the 1980s arose because of the need to account for any improved outcome in a subject arising simply due to the increased attention being afforded them by virtue of being involved in research ('Hawthorne' effect). Potentially it could be unclear whether any physiological or behavioural response in a subject was due to the drug treatment or just due to being involved in an experiment. A placebo is an inert substance with no known physiological effects but which looks the same as the active drug. A placebo is given to control subjects taking part in drug trials so that any changes due to the Hawthorne effect can be identified and compared with any 'real' changes due to the drug itself.

Exercise 8

Before moving on, read the following description of an experimental study to check your understanding of the terms that have been introduced so far. This intervention study was carried out in 1985 by a research unit based at the University of London. The group wanted to address the question: 'Does social support given to women during pregnancy improve women's satisfaction after delivery and infant birth weight?'

Oakley A (1985) Social support in pregnancy: the 'soft' way to increase birthweight? *Social Science & Medicine.* **21**, 11: 1259–68.

A total of 509 women agreed to take part in the study over a 15-month period. They were randomly allocated into two groups. One group received social support by one of four midwives who visited the women at home throughout the women's pregnancy and offered them various forms of practical and emotional help when required. The other group of subjects received no special support, only the existing maternity care provisions. Women in both groups had previously given birth to one low-birthweight baby. Women's satisfaction and infant birthweight were evaluated after delivery using obstetric case note information from the hospitals and by sending the women a questionnaire to complete and return.

1. What is the independent variable in this study?
2. What are the dependent variables in this study?
3. Other than the independent variables, what other variables could influence the outcome of this study? What are these variables collectively known as?
4. What is the name given to the group who received standard care?

Selection of subjects and random allocation to groups

An experiment is carried out on a sample of subjects. Sampling is the selection of a representative portion of the population. It is important that the sample is a true representation of the population. The population should be clearly defined using strict criteria decided upon during the planning of an experiment. A researcher should avoid working with an atypical or biased sample and ensure that the sample represents the heterogenetic range within the population. Clearly the larger the sample the more likely it is to accurately represent the population. However, in experimental research time, costs and availability of subjects mean that sample sizes have to be relatively small. *Sampling* is a complex topic that is covered in detail in the Trent Focus research volume

Statistical Analysis in Primary Care, Chapter 2 'Sampling'. It is essential that any researcher undertaking experimental research needs to ensure that their sample is selected in an unbiased way. *Random sampling* is the most commonly used method of ensuring that an unbiased sample is chosen. The term random in this context means 'by chance' rather than 'haphazard'.

The process of randomly allocating subjects to the control or experimental group can be done in many different ways; for example by tossing a coin or using a table of random numbers. In her 1990 study of social support in pregnancy, Oakley outlines the process and problems she encountered:

> 'Randomisation was done by the midwives telephoning us at TCRU with the names of women who had agreed to take part. The study 'secretary' had sheets of allocations derived from a table of random numbers and she entered each woman in order, then informing the midwife of the result of the allocation.'

The midwives in this study, however, were often unhappy about this process because the women could not choose whether they received extra support and also because the midwives were concerned about those women who they felt needed more support being allocated to the control group. Hence there was conflict between the midwives' professional opinions and the need to maintain scientific rigour.

Informed consent

(This topic is covered in more detail in the Trent Focus research volume *Developing Research in Primary Care*, Chapter 3 'Ethical considerations in research'.) It is important for the researcher to be aware of how informed consent specifically relates to experimental research. Prospective subjects must have adequate information about the potential health costs and benefits to themselves before taking part in the experiment, so that they can make an informed choice about whether or not they wish to take part. This principle of informed consent is perhaps more pertinent in experimental research (though necessary in other types of research as well) because subjects are exposed to an intervention such as a new drug or procedure. The intervention may be beneficial to the individual, but it may be harmful, if only in terms of costs in time, money or inconvenience. Informed consent can be sought at different times in the experimental protocol. The issues relating to these different possibilities are discussed in Oakley's 'Who's afraid of the Randomised Controlled Trial?' (1990). Figure 2.1 shows one of these options: perhaps the most popular choice. Informed consent is gained immediately following the selection of the subjects. The process of random allocation to control and experimental groups is carried out on those who agree to continue with the experiment.

The amount of information given to the subject varies depending on the research question. In some experiments, giving too much information can invalidate the study.

Experimental designs

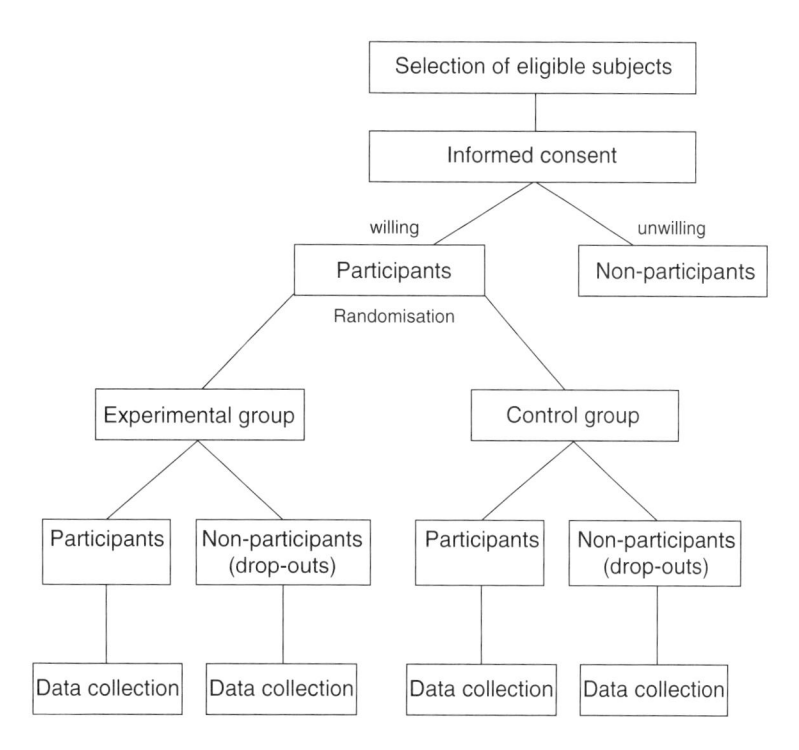

Figure 2.1 Informed consent.

Example

Kerrigan D D et al. (1993) Who's afraid of informed consent? *BMJ*. **306**: 298–300.

> 'Patients were simply told that we were aware that emotions could influence how they reacted to illness and were asked to participate in a survey investigating their response to hospital admissions for minor surgery. They were not aware that they were taking part in a randomised comparison of two different information sheets, as this would have invalidated the study, which received ethical approval from the Royal Hallamshire Hospital ethical committee.'

Exercise 9

Test your understanding of this section by answering the following questions:

1. Why is it important to randomly select subjects for an experimental study?
2. Why should subjects be randomly allocated to the experimental and control groups in an experiment?

Summary

When reading literature that reports on a study using an experimental design, or when planning your own experiment, you should assess the following in the methods:

- validity and reliability of the dependent variable
- standardisation of the techniques and protocol (independent variable)
- control of confounding variables.

Where these haven't been considered in the methods, they should be taken into account when interpreting and discussing the results as shown in the example below.

Example

Forster and Young (1996) Specialist nurse support for patients with stroke in the community: a randomised controlled trial. *BMJ.* **312**: 1642–46.

> 'This was a pragmatic randomised trial with a heterogeneous population including patients with aphasia, cognitive impairment, and diverse ethnic backgrounds. The study needed widespread local support, and therefore knowledge of the trial's objectives may have raised other community staff's awareness of psychosocial problems related to stroke. Moreover, intermittent professional contact with the specialist nurses will have further emphasised this effect. Inevitably there will have been contact between the two groups of patients with stroke at day centres, stroke clubs, or local community gatherings. All these potentially confounding factors would have been in the direction of reducing the measured effectiveness of the trial. Lastly, during the 12 months, other significant life events – such as new physical illness or bereavement – took place and are likely to have influenced the psychological state and social functioning of the patients; we found no evidence, however, that such adverse events were more frequent in one or other group.'

Research designs

This section of the chapter will introduce you to a number of common research designs. The previous section described features that needed to be considered when designing experiments. In an ideal world, all experiments would be designed so that they were fully randomised and controlled with no confounding variables! In reality, of course, this is not often possible to achieve, and research designs with less rigour are chosen because opportunities arise to obtain data, and time, financial constraints or transitory 'ideal' circumstances mean that randomisation or pre-testing are not feasible. As long as the limitations of the experiment are recognised and the effect on the validity of the results acknowledged, then some reduced rigour is accepted.

Experimental designs **37**

Within-subject designs

Single-subject designs

The simplest possible design is to apply an intervention to a single subject and measure the response. Say you suspected that a drug was causing a patient's temperature to increase, you could investigate this further by monitoring the temperature to establish a baseline – let's call this control Condition A – then a dose of the drug is given and the temperature continues to be monitored (experimental Condition B). If a rise in temperature coincides with the time that the drug is known to take to enter the bloodstream then you may surmise that the drug is raising body temperature. This is represented schematically in Figure 2.2.

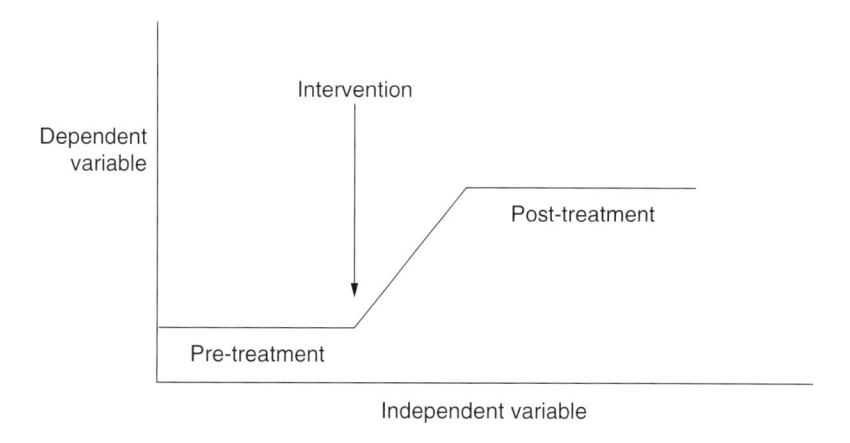

Figure 2.2 Schematic diagram of a single-subject experimental design.

Following on from this, you could then continue to monitor temperature as the drug was eliminated from the body, then re-administer the drug when the temperature had returned to baseline levels. This then becomes an ABAB design. Studies of single subjects are often referred to as 'n of one' studies.

Exercise 10

Continue the graph in Figure 2.2 to show what you might expect to see in an ABAB design.

A stable baseline (Condition A) is essential in single-subject designs since, if this is fluctuating considerably, it is impossible to assess the influence of Condition B. The baseline measurement should be made for a long enough time for the researchers to be confident that a baseline level has been determined and is reliable. The validity will be improved if the intervention is applied a number of times (i.e. ABABAB).

These single-subject designs are important in health sciences because in clinical practice settings healthcare workers are always dealing with individual patients who are unique in the way their condition progresses and the treatment they require. Hence when assessing the results of a particular therapy in a single case where these designs are acceptable, the problem arises when a researcher wishes to generalise the results to a wider population. Single-subject experiments provide useful preliminary data, which can then be extended to larger group studies in which the treatment can be evaluated.

Subject group designs

A group design involves a group of subjects in an experiment. Each subject is exposed to more than one experimental condition. Box 2.3 shows a design in which subjects receive a standard treatment (control condition) and then a new treatment.

Box 2.3		
Subject	**Week 1**	**Week 2**
1	standard treatment	new treatment
2	standard treatment	new treatment
3	standard treatment	new treatment
4	standard treatment	new treatment

Exercise 11

There is a major flaw in this design. Can you think what it is?

Consider if something happened in Week 1 which affected the dependent variable in one or more of the subjects which did not occur in Week 2. For example, say the dependent variable was body temperature and the independent variable was a new drug treatment or the standard drug treatment (control treatment). If all the subjects, unknown to them or the researchers, were exposed to an infection during Week 1, this is likely to raise body temperature. Our baseline measurement would be inaccurate and the comparison with temperature measured during the new treatment period in Week 2 would be invalid. The term *maturation* refers to incidents such as the infection which may arise during the course of an experiment, other examples include policy changes, practice effects and developmental changes. The longer an experiment continues the more likely it is that external events might influence the dependent variable. This can be overcome by *balancing* the design as shown in Box 2.4. This is also called a *cross-over design*.

Now any unknown confounding variable affecting the subjects in Week 1 will be spread across the treatments and will have less influence on the results. An extension of this type of design is known as a *repeated measures* design: that is, subjects repeat their performance but under slightly different conditions. More than two conditions are allowed

Box 2.4		
Subject	**Week 1**	**Week 2**
1	standard treatment	new treatment
2	new treatment	standard treatment
3	standard treatment	new treatment
4	new treatment	standard treatment

in repeated measures designs, but it is worth bearing in mind that subjects understandably get bored and tired when participating in long experiments. These fatigue effects are more important in within-subject designs, so it is more likely that subjects will drop out of the study or exhibit reduced performance. When subjects are lost from an experiment they are known as *drop-outs*.

So what are the advantages of using within-subject designs? There is a large variability between subjects both in their physiological responses and behaviour; this source of variation is reduced by using the same subjects in an experiment. Unfortunately it is often not possible to use the same subjects because in many experiments exposure to one intervention means that they cannot participate again. An example would be giving information to a subject about symptoms they may experience on returning home after surgery to see whether it relieved anxiety – a subject could not undertake this twice! In these circumstances a between-subject design is used.

Between-subject designs

In these designs, different subjects are used for the control and intervention groups. In the previous section we talked about random allocation of subjects to ensure that extraneous variables are spread equally between the groups. Variation in subject characteristics should be equal for control and treatment groups. The characteristics of all the groups should always be compared, particularly for age, sex and previous exposure to any experience, which might influence the dependent variable. The pre-test values of the dependent variable should be comparable between the groups. Random allocation can eradicate what is termed *systematic bias*, since every person has exactly the same chance of being selected for the intervention or control groups, although chance difference may arise. In Box 2.5, which is part of a table in a published paper reporting the effect on mood of lowering cholesterol concentration, you can see how randomly allocating the subjects to the control and treatment group has led to remarkably comparable baseline measures in the groups. A more complex procedure to optimise baseline matching between groups of subjects is called stratification or *stratified sampling*. Stratification may be based on a variety of attributes, such as age, gender and occupation.

Example

Wardle J et al. (1996) Randomised placebo controlled trial of effect on mood of lowering cholesterol concentration. *BMJ.* **313**: 75–78.

Box 2.5		
	Simvastatin 20 mg or 40 mg (n=334)	Placebo control (n=157)
Mean age (years)	63.3	63.8
Mean total cholesterol (mmol/l)	7.0	6.9
Mean low-density lipoprotein cholesterol (mmol/l)	4.8	4.7
Mean low-density lipoprotein cholesterol (mmol/l)	1.17	1.14
Mean triglycerides (mmol/l)	2.52	2.59

Matched-pair designs

The *matched-pair* design also uses different subjects in the groups. Random allocation does not guarantee that the groups are equivalent, rather that the chances are they won't be different. In matched-pair designs the researcher first identifies characteristics that might influence the outcome and then selects subjects who are matched for these characteristics; matching for age and sex is common. Random allocation to the control or treatment groups occurs after the matching procedure.

Example

Forster A and Young J (1996) Specialist nurse support for patients with stroke in the community: a randomised controlled trial. *BMJ.* **312**: 1642–46.

> 'Once recruited, the patients were stratified by whether they had been admitted to hospital or stayed at home, by level of social activities before their stroke (Frenchay activities index, categories 0–10, 11–30, 31–45), and by functional ability (the Barthel index, categories 0–9, 10–14, 15–19, 20).'

The allocation of subjects to treatment or control groups in health research raises a number of ethical issues. In particular a researcher may be concerned when a subject is denied a potentially beneficial treatment if allocated to the control group (remember the midwives' concerns in the earlier section).

Experimental designs

Exercise 12

From the extracts taken from the following research papers, decide which type of experimental design has been used in these studies.

1. Bainton D *et al.* (1982) Pads and pants for urinary incontinence.
   51 female patients, incontinent of urine, were asked to compare two different combinations of pants and pads used in ambulatory management of their incontinence.
2. Kerrigan D D *et al.* (1993) Who's afraid of informed consent?
   Pre-operative anxiety assessed before and after patients were randomly allocated an information sheet containing either simple or detailed descriptions of possible post-operative complications.
3. Forster A and Young J (1996) Specialist nurse support for patients with stroke in the community.
   To evaluate whether specialist nurse visits enhance the social integration and perceived health of patients with stroke or alleviate stress in carers in long-term stroke.

Variations in experimental designs

Pre-test–post-test designs

In the classical experiment the dependent variable is measured both before and after the intervention or treatment in a control or experimental group (see Figure 2.2). The pre-test measurement gives what is often called a *baseline* measure of the dependent variable. This allows two comparisons to be made in the analysis. Firstly, the change from baseline in the control and experimental groups and secondly, a comparison of post-test measures of the dependent variable in the control and experimental groups. This gives more information about the possible cause–effect relationship of the independent and dependent variables.

Example

In a trial studying the effects of weight-bearing exercise on bone in post-menopausal women, McMurdo *et al.* (1997) compared a group taking only calcium supplements with a group taking calcium supplements and exercise. The bone mineral content was measured at two sites in the forearm and in the lumbar spine, both at entry into the study (baseline or pre-test measure) and after two years. Box 2.6 shows some of the results they obtained.

Pre-test bone density has been subtracted from the post-test values to allow a percentage change in bone density to be calculated. This percentage change can then be compared

Box 2.6 Change in bone mineral content and density over two years of study

Site	Mean % change	
	Calcium group (n=48)	Calcium and exercise (n=44)
Ultradistal forearm	−2.6	1.14
Distal forearm	−1.38	−2.18
Lumbar spine	−2.65	−0.91

Box 2.7

Experimental group 1	pre-test measurement	intervention	post-test measurement
Experimental group 2	pre-test measurement	intervention	post-test measurement
Stage:	1	2	3

in the control (calcium only) and experimental (calcium and exercise) groups. Statistical analysis would then show whether the percentage changes and the comparisons between groups were statistically significant.

Post-test only designs

Sometimes it is not appropriate to do a pre-test measurement and just post-test measurements are carried out in control and treatment groups. The post-test results from the two groups are then compared. This is a weaker design and difference between groups may have been present before the intervention.

Exercise 13

Read Extract 2 on page 31 describing West Berkshire perineal management trial. It is easy to see why a pre-test measurement was not possible in this trial! Can you identify all the post-test measurements (outcome measures) made by the researchers mentioned in this abstract.

Number of dependent variables

It is also permissible to measure more than one dependent variable, for example in a pressure-sore experiment, the researcher might want to measure number of sores, grade of sores and size of sores. This increases and complicates the statistical analysis of the data, however, and subjects may get fatigued if too many measurements are made on them.

Experimental designs

Number of independent variables

It was stated in the introduction that the researcher should not be tempted to try to answer too many research questions within one experiment. This implies that one should not manipulate more than one independent variable at a time. Sometimes a researcher does want to study the individual and combined effects of two or more independent variables. Such designs are called *factorial designs*. If the two independent variables have two levels (see the example below) the design is called a 2 ×2 factorial design and four groups of subjects would be needed. Factorial designs permit the testing of multiple hypotheses in a single experiment.

Example

Melnyck *et al.* (1994) studied the effect of receiving or not receiving two types of information on mothers' and children's ability to cope with an unplanned childhood hospitalisation. The design is shown in Table 2.2, with the number of subjects receiving neither, one, or both sets of information shown in the cells:

Table 2.2

		Child behavioural information	
		Received	Did not receive
Parental role information	Received	27	22
	Did not receive	26	23

The two independent variables are child behavioural information and parental role information and there are two levels of measurement for the two independent variables: receiving and not receiving the information.

Community trials

A community trial is an experimental study conducted on a whole community rather than on a small sample. The best example to use is the study carried out by the British government on the fluoridation of water. In 1955, the British government fluoridated the water supply in Watford, Kilmarnock and parts of Anglesey and measured the proportion of children with caries-free teeth. In Holyhead (fluoridated) and Bodafon (non-fluoridated) the proportions, before fluoridation, were 13% and 12% respectively. Ten years later, after fluoridation in Holyhead, they did a post-test measurement of the proportion of children with caries-free teeth. The proportions were 40% for Holyhead and 14% for Bodafon.

Summary

When planning an experiment or reading about experimental research you need to consider whether the design chosen is appropriate for the research question posed. A researcher may choose:

- a between-subject, within-subject or matched-pair design
- a pre-test–post-test design or a post-test only design
- a factorial design, when the effect of individual or combined effects of more than one independent variable are to be investigated.

Benefits and limitations of experimental research

Introduction

The advantages and limitations of experimental research have been implied throughout the previous sections of this chapter. This section will provide a summary of the main benefits and limitations of experimental research and when this method should be used. The special considerations relating specifically to human experimentation can be grouped as factors relating to causality, validity, and humanity and ethics.

Causal relationships between variables

The previous sections have identified three features that characterise a true experiment. In experimental research, the researcher:

- manipulates the experimental situation by systematically varying the independent variable and measuring the response in the dependent variable
- introduces some control over the experimental situation by eliminating the influence of variables other than the independent and dependent variables
- randomly selects and allocates the subjects to a control group (no treatment or standard treatment) and experimental group (treatment).

Experimental research is the most powerful method for inferring causal relationships between variables. This is because the researcher has eliminated all possible factors that could account for a change in one or more outcome (or dependent) variable(s) other than the influence of one or more explanatory (or independent) variable(s).

Sometimes it is not possible to fulfil all these requirements, so, for example, it may be unethical to have a control group or it may not be possible to carry out randomisation. Such experiments are then called *quasi-experiments*. In Woolf's hierarchy of evidence (1990) (Box 2.8), well-designed, randomised controlled trials (true experiments) are

Experimental designs

> **Box 2.8 Woolf's hierarchy of evidence**
>
> I   well-designed randomised controlled trials
> II-1   other types of trial; well-designed controlled trial without randomisation; quasi-experiments
> II-2   well-designed cohort (prospective) study, preferably from more than one centre
> II-3   well-designed case–control (retrospective) study, preferably from several centres
> III   large differences from comparisons between time and/or places with or without intervention
> IV   opinions of respected authorities based on clinical experience; descriptive studies and reports of expert committees

considered the most useful evidence for establishing causal relationships with experiments with less control (quasi-experiments) lower down the hierarchy.

Some caution should be exercised when inferring cause–effect relationships between the independent and dependent variables. Few non-experimental studies are so well designed that the researchers are 100% confident that the change in the independent variable *caused* the change in the dependent variable. More often researchers acknowledge an *association* or *relationship* between the variables; causality is only proven after many studies have been carried out.

Internal and external validity

Of all the research methods, experimental research is said to have high internal validity because it is a more controlled approach. Any factor that interferes with the design or implementation of an experiment potentially threatens the internal validity of that experiment. To check whether an experiment has internal validity you should ask the question: 'Are the changes in the dependent variable only due to the intervention (the independent variable) and not due to other factors?'

Exercise 14

Think back over what we have already covered and, before reading further, write down some of the features of experimental design that ensure high internal validity.

Some of the factors you might have written down are:

1. Control of confounding variables.
2. Reliable instruments.
3. Appropriate choice of independent and dependent variables.
4. Random selection to groups.
5. Standardisation of protocol.
6. Minimising factors such as maturation, history and mortality.

Internal validity ——— External validity

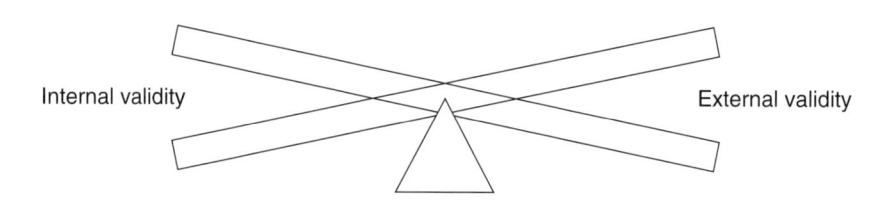

Figure 2.3

Exercise 15
Would a quasi-experiment have a higher or lower internal validity than a true experiment? Explain why and add 'true experiment' and 'quasi-experiment' to Figure 2.3.

Some researchers believe that the true experiment produces an unreal situation because of the strict control over conditions, a situation that would not normally occur in everyday life, hence results from experiments are not generalisable to the wider population. External validity answers the question: 'Can the results be generalised to the wider population?'

External validity can be improved by *replicating* experiments: that is, repeating the experiment under similar conditions. Researchers might wish to use a slightly modified research tool, a different setting or subjects with slightly different characteristics; all of these changes would increase the generalisability of the research and improve the external validity.

Humanity and ethics

The researcher using human subjects in experimental research may frequently come across situations where ethics and considerations for fellow human beings conflict with the strict control required in the methodology. Experiments involving human subjects who do not behave as predictably as inanimate objects, and are less compliant, require some special considerations. These are listed below:

- the need to protect human rights
- the importance of preventing unnecessary suffering and risk to subjects
- subjects should give *informed* consent, even though this may affect the results and conclusions
- the need for subjects to comply with protocol while recognising the importance of 'free will'
- being objective when studying fellow human beings whom the researcher might like or dislike
- difficulty of measuring dependent variables when they concern subjective and complex emotions or behaviours, e.g. stress, pain, intelligence
- ensuring all variables are held constant except the independent variable(s)
- withholding a possible beneficial treatment from clients in the control group

Experimental designs

- subjects' behaviour may change when they know they are being studied ('Hawthorne effect')
- artificiality of human behaviour in experiments compared to 'real life'.

Some of these issues have been discussed in other parts of the chapter. Ethical issues need to be considered when planning and implementing any research. This topic is covered in the Trent Focus research volume *Developing Research in Primary Care*, Chapter 3 'Ethical considerations in research'.

Exercise 16

Check your understanding of this section by listing three advantages and three disadvantages of experimental research.

When to use experimental designs

We have considered some of the advantages and disadvantages of experimental research throughout this chapter and by now you should have some idea of when to use an experimental approach to research. If your research question is fairly specific and you want to compare the effectiveness of one or more treatments (or interventions), then the experimental approach is the best to use. Other methods such as observational, surveys and qualitative approaches should be used when the research aims are broader and an overview of opinions or behaviour is required. The validity of the research will be threatened if an experiment is badly designed or inappropriate for the research question, e.g. if it is not possible to impose the necessary control and randomisation which are fundamental to experimental design, perhaps for ethical or practical reasons. Reading through studies that have used an experimental approach will help you to understand the type of research questions requiring an experimental approach. Examples of a range of experimental studies can be found in the reference list at the end of this chapter.

Answers to exercises

Exercise 1

1. Pressure-sore grade.
2. Mattress type.

Exercise 2

'Our study was designed to determine the effectiveness in pressure-sore prevention of a new interface pressure-decreasing mattress.'

Exercise 3

There is no difference in the effectiveness in pressure-sore prevention of the new interface pressure-decreasing mattress and the standard mattress.

Exercise 4

Potentially there are many sources of systematic error; however, some you may have identified are:

- uncalibrated sphygmomanometer which always reads higher or lower than the true pressure
- not taking account of the mercury meniscus when reading the pressure
- sphygmomanometer not zeroed.

Exercise 5

Feedback in text.

Exercise 6

- psychological condition
- age
- sex
- mobility
- nursing/medical care
- nutrition
- medical/surgical intervention

All these factors are potentially confounding variables. The authors have said in the abstract, however, that both groups were treated using a standard protocol for the prevention of pressure sores and that the two groups were similar in patient characteristics and pressure-sore risk factors.

Exercise 7

Either of these treatments could be considered to be the 'standard' policy. This will depend on the individual midwives' and obstetricians' clinical judgement.

Experimental designs

Description of control group:

Extract 1: nursed on a standard mattress
Extract 2: allocated simple information sheet
Extract 3: liberal or restrictive policy.

Exercise 8

1. Social support.
2. Women's satisfaction and infant birthweight.
3. All women had given birth to one low-birthweight baby. There are many *confounding* variables in a study of this kind which is why a qualitative approach is often preferred for this type of research question. Some of the confounding variables you might have identified are:
   - some mothers may have received social support from other sources, e.g. relatives and friends
   - women in the control group may have felt more supported just because they were taking part in a research project.
4. The standard care group is a *control group*.

Exercise 9

1. Random selection is important to avoid selecting a biased or atypical sample from a population.
2. To increase the likelihood that the control and experimental groups will be comparable in terms of subject characteristics and baseline measures.

Exercise 10

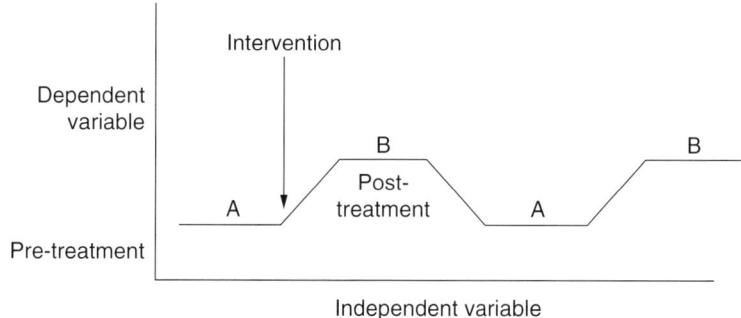

Exercise 11

Feedback in text.

Exercise 12

1. Within-subject design.
2. Between-subject design.
3. Between-subject design.

Exercise 13

1. Dependent variables (outcome measures).
2. Perineal and labial tears.
3. Neonatal state, maternal pain and urinary symptoms at ten days and at three months.
4. Likelihood of resumption of sexual intercourse within one month.

Exercise 14

Feedback in text.

Exercise 15

Lower internal validity; because there are less strict controls in the design of quasi-experiments.

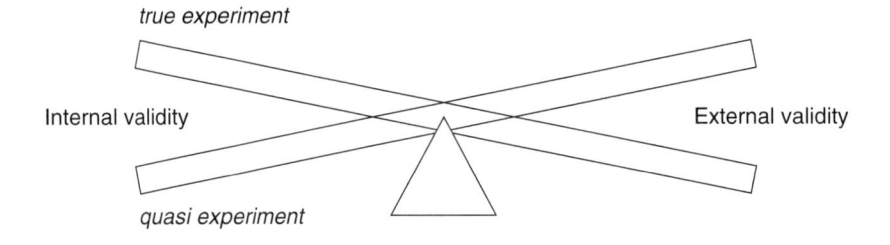

Exercise 16

Advantages: high internal validity; researcher has more control over the research; specific relationships between variables can be studied.

Disadvantages: Low external validity; only consider a relatively small number of variables; ethical and practical difficulties of imposing control and randomisation.

References

Bainton D, Blannin J B and Shepherd A M (1982) Pads and pants for urinary incontinence. *BMJ.* **285**: 419–20.

Boore J R P et al. (1978) *Prescription for Recovery: the effect of pre-operative preparation of surgical patients on post-operative stress, recovery and infection.* Royal College of Nursing, London.

Clegg F (1994) *Simple Statistics* (12e). Cambridge University Press, Cambridge.

Forster A and Young J (1996) Specialist nurse support for patients with stroke in the community: a randomised controlled trial. *BMJ.* **312**: 1642–46.

Hofman A, Geelkerken R H, Wille J, Hamming J J and Breslau P J (1994) Pressure sores and pressure-decreasing mattresses: controlled clinical trial. *Lancet.* **343**: 568–71.

Kerrigan D D, Thevasagayam R S, Woods T O et al. (1993) Who's afraid of informed consent? *BMJ.* **306**: 298–300.

McMurdo M E T, Mole P A and Paterson C R (1997) Controlled trial of weight-bearing exercise in older women in relation to bone density and falls. *BMJ.* **314**: 569.

Melnyck B M (1994) Coping with unplanned childhood hospitalization. Effects of informational interventions on mothers and children. *Nursing Res.* **43**: 50–55.

Melzack R et al. (1975) The McGill pain questionnaire: major properties and scoring methods. *Pain.* **1**: 277–99.

Melzack R, Abbott F V, Zackon W, Mulder D S and Davis M W L (1987) Pain on a surgical ward: a survey of the duration and intensity of pain and the effectiveness of medication. *Pain.* **29**: 67–72.

Oakley A (1985) Social support in pregnancy: the 'soft' way to increase birthweight? *Social Science & Medicine.* **21**: 11: 1259–68.

Oakley A (1990) Who's afraid of the Randomised Controlled Trial? In: H Roberts (ed) *Women's Health Counts.* Routledge, London.

O'Brian D and Davison M (1994) Blood pressure measurement: rational and ritual actions. *Br. J. Nursing.* **3**: 393–96.

Roe B H (1990) Study of the effects of education on patients' knowledge and acceptance of indwelling urethral catheters. *J. Adv. Nursing.* **15**: 223–31.

Rose G, Hamilton P J S et al. (1978) A randomised controlled trial of the effect on middle-aged men of advice to stop smoking. *J. Epid. & Comm. Health.* **32**: 275–81.

Sleep J, Grant A, Garcia J, Elbourne D, Spencer J and Chalmers I (1984) West Berkshire perineal management trial. *BMJ.* **289**: 587–90.

Wardle J *et al.* (1996) Randomised placebo-controlled trial of effect on mood of lowering cholesterol concentration. *BMJ.* **313**: 75–78.

Wilson-Barnet J (1991) The Experiment: Is it worthwhile? *Int. J. Nurs. Stud.* **28**: 77–87.

Woolf S H *et al.* (1990) Assessing the clinical effectiveness of preventive manoeuvres: analytical principles and systematic methods in reviewing evidence and developing clinical practice recommendations. *J. Clin. Epidemiology.* **43**: 891–905.

Further reading

Polgar S and Thomas S A (1995) *Introduction to research in the health sciences* (3e). Churchill Livingstone, Edinburgh.

Polit D F and Hungler B P (1995) *Nursing Research – Principles and Methods* (5e). J B Lippincott & Co., Philadelphia.

Rose G and Hamilton P J S (1978) A randomised controlled trial of the effect on middle-aged men of advice to stop smoking. *J. Epidem. & Comm. Health.* **32**: 275–81.

Sapsford R and Abbott P (1992) *Research Methods for Nurses and the Caring Professions.* Oxford University Press, Oxford.

Self-completing glossary

Create your own glossary of terms as you work through the chapter.

baseline
between-subject design
bias
carry-over effects
community trials
confounding variables
content validity
control
control group
dependent variables
double-blind
external validity
extraneous variables
face validity
fatigue

Experimental designs

independent variables
informed consent
internal validity
intervention
hypothesis
matched-pair design
mortality
multi-centred randomised controlled trials
null hypothesis
potency
pilot study
population
post-test only designs
pre-test–post-test designs
qualitative
quasi-experiments
random sampling
randomised clinical (controlled) trials (rcts)
reliability
repeated measures
replicating
reproducible
sample
sampling
single-subject designs
standardise
systematic bias
systematic error
validity
variables
within-subject designs

CHAPTER THREE

Qualitative research

Beverley Hancock

Introduction

A starting point in trying to understand the collection of information for research purposes is that there are broadly two approaches: quantitative research and qualitative research. Early forms of research originated in the natural sciences such as biology, chemistry, physics, geology etc., and was concerned with investigating elements which we could observe and measure in some way. Such observations and measurements can be made objectively and repeated by other researchers. This process is referred to as 'quantitative' research.

Much later, along came researchers working in the social sciences: for example psychology, sociology and anthropology. They were interested in studying human behaviour and the social world inhabited by human beings. They found increasing difficulty in trying to explain human behaviour in simply measurable terms. Measurements tell us how often or how many people behave in a certain way but they do not adequately answer the question 'why?'. Research which attempts to increase our understanding of why things are the way they are in our social world and why people act the ways they do is 'qualitative' research.

The purpose of this chapter is to enable primary healthcare professionals with little or no previous experience of research to gain a basic understanding of qualitative research and the potential for this type of research in primary healthcare.

The chapter begins with a general introduction into the nature of qualitative research. This includes identification of the strengths and weaknesses of qualitative research in a brief comparison with quantitative research. This is followed by short descriptions of the main qualitative approaches and ways of collecting information. Clear and practical guidance is then provided on techniques for analysing and presenting information. Theoretical information is reinforced through exercises and examples drawn from primary healthcare.

The aims of the chapter are as follows:

- to provide the reader with a basic understanding of qualitative research

- to equip the reader with sufficient information to appreciate how qualitative research is undertaken
- to enable prospective researchers to consider the appropriateness of a qualitative approach to their chosen field of investigation
- to provide practitioners contemplating or undertaking qualitative research for the first time with guidance on the collection and analysis of data.

The nature of qualitative research

Qualitative research is concerned with developing explanations of social phenomena. That is to say, it aims to help us to understand the world in which we live and why things are the way they are. It is concerned with the social aspects of our world and seeks to answer questions about:

- why people behave the way they do
- how opinions and attitudes are formed
- how people are affected by the events that go on around them
- how and why cultures have developed in the way they have
- the differences between social groups.

Qualitative research is concerned with finding the answers to questions which begin with: Why? How? and In what way? Quantitative research, on the other hand, is more concerned with questions like: How much? How many? How often? and To what extent? Further features of qualitative research and how it differs from quantitative research are as follows:

1. Qualitative research is concerned with the opinions, experiences and feelings of individuals producing subjective data.
2. Qualitative research describes social phenomena as they occur naturally, with no attempt made to manipulate the situation under study, as is the case with experimental quantitative research.
3. Understanding of a situation is gained through an holistic perspective, whereas quantitative research depends on the ability to identify a set of variables.
4. Data are used to develop concepts and theories which help us to understand the social world. This is an inductive approach to the development of theory. Quantitative research is deductive in that it tests theories which have already been proposed.
5. Qualitative data are collected through direct encounters with individuals, through one-to-one interviews or group interviews or by observation. Data collection is time-consuming.
6. The intensive and time-consuming nature of data collection necessitates the use of small samples.
7. Different sampling techniques are used. In quantitative research, sampling seeks to demonstrate representativeness of findings through random selection of subjects.

Table 3.1 Comparison of qualitative and quantitative research terms

Qualitative research	Quantitative research
Subjective	Objective
Holistic	Reductionist
Phenomenological	Scientific
Anti-positivist	Positivist
Descriptive	Experimental
Naturalistic	Contrived
Inductive	Deductive

Qualitative sampling techniques are concerned with seeking information from specific groups and subgroups in the population.

8. Criteria used to assess reliability and validity differ from those used in quantitative research.
9. A review of textbooks reveals a variety of terms used to describe the nature of qualitative and quantitative research. Some of the common terms are listed in Table 3.1.

Each of the various features of qualitative research may be viewed as a strength or a weakness. This depends on the original purpose of the research. For example, one common criticism levied at qualitative research is that the results of a study may not be generalisable to a larger population because the sample group was small and the subjects were not chosen randomly. But the original research question may have sought insight into a specific subgroup of the population, not the general population because the subgroup is 'special' or different from the general population and that specialness is the focus of the research. The small sample may have been necessary because very few subjects were available such as is the case with some ethnic groups or patient groups suffering from a rare condition. In such studies, generalisability of the findings to a wider, more diverse population is not an aim.

Exercise 1

Look at the research projects listed below. In which projects would you expect to see a qualitative approach used and in which projects would you expect to see a quantitative approach? Why?

1. A comparison of the effectiveness of drug A versus drug B in the treatment of migraine.
2. An exploration of the role of the practice manager in the primary healthcare team: a study of four practices.
3. A descriptive study of school nurses' experiences of dealing with boys who have eating disorders.
4. A national survey of patients' knowledge of the causes of heart disease.

Qualitative research designs

In this section, four major types of qualitative research design are outlined. They are:

- phenomenology
- ethnography
- grounded theory
- case study.

Another common research design is the survey. Surveys can be either qualitative or quantitative in their approach to data collection. A description of qualitative surveys can be found in the appropriate chapter.

Phenomenology

The terminology used by different authors can be very confusing and the use of the term *phenomenology* is one example. In the first section of this chapter, phenomenology was listed as one of the terms used to describe qualitative research generally. However, it is also used to describe a particular type of qualitative research.

Phenomenology literally means the study of phenomena. It is a way of describing something that exists as part of the world in which we live. Phenomena may be events, situations, experiences or concepts. We are surrounded by many phenomena, which we are aware of but don't fully understand. Our lack of understanding of these phenomena may exist because the phenomenon has not been overtly described and explained, or because our understanding of the impact it makes may be unclear. For example, we know that lots of people are carers. But what does 'caring' actually mean and what is it like to be a carer?

Back pain is another example. Correlation studies may tell us about the types of people who experience back pain and the apparent causes. Randomised controlled trials of drugs compare the effectiveness of one analgesia against another. But what is it actually like to live with back pain? What are the effects on peoples' lives? What problems does it cause? A phenomenological study might explore, for example, the effect that back pain has on sufferers' relationships with other people by describing the strain it can cause in marriages, or the effect on children of having a disabled parent.

Phenomenological research begins with the acknowledgement that there is a gap in our understanding and that clarification or illumination will be of benefit. Phenomenological research will not necessarily provide definitive explanations, but it does raise awareness and increases insight.

Ethnography

Ethnography has a background in anthropology. The term means 'portrait of a people' and it is a methodology for descriptive studies of cultures and peoples. The cultural parameter is that the people under investigation have something in common. Examples of parameters include:

- geographical – a particular region or country
- religious
- tribal
- shared experience.

In healthcare settings, researchers may choose an ethnographic approach because the cultural parameter is suspected of affecting the population's response to care or treatment. For example, cultural rules about contact between males and females may contribute to reluctance of women from an Asian subgroup to take up cervical screening. Ethnography helps healthcare professionals to develop cultural awareness and sensitivity and enhances the provision and quality of care for people from all cultures.

Ethnographic studies entail extensive fieldwork by the researcher. Data collection techniques include both formal and informal interviewing (often interviewing individuals on several occasions) and participant observation. Because of this, ethnography is extremely time-consuming as it involves the researcher spending long periods of time in the field.

Analysis of data adopts an 'emic' approach. This means that the researcher attempts to interpret data from the perspective of the population under study. The results are expressed as though they were being expressed by the subjects themselves, often using local language and terminology to describe phenomena. For example, a researcher may explore behaviour which we traditionally in the westernised medical world would describe as mental illness. However, within the population under study, the behaviour may not be characterised as illness but as something else – as evidence that the individual is 'blessed' or 'gifted' in some way.

Ethnographic research can be problematic when researchers are not sufficiently familiar with the social mores of the people being studied or with their language. Interpretation from an 'etic' perspective – an outsider perspective – may be a misinterpretation causing confusion. For this reason, the ethnographic researcher usually returns to the field to check his interpretations with informants, thereby validating the data before presenting the findings.

Grounded theory

This methodology originated with Glaser and Strauss (1967) and their work on the interactions between healthcare professionals and dying patients. The main feature is the development of new theory through the collection and analysis of data about a phenomenon. It goes beyond phenomenology because the explanations that emerge are genuinely *new* knowledge and are used to develop new theories about a phenomenon. In healthcare settings the new theories can be applied, enabling us to approach existing problems in a new way, e.g. our approaches to health promotion or the provision of care.

One example of grounded theory with which many of us are familiar is theory about the grief process. Researchers observed that people who were bereaved progressed through a series of stages and that each stage was characterised by certain responses: denial, anger, acceptance and resolution. This is not a new phenomenon, people have been going through these stages for as long as society has existed, but the research formally acknowledged and described the experience. Now we use our knowledge of the grief process, new knowledge derived from grounded theory, to understand the experience of bereavement and to help the bereaved to come to terms with their loss. We recognise when a person is having difficulty coming to terms with loss because we use the knowledge to recognise signs of 'abnormal' grief and can offer help.

Various data-collection techniques are used to develop grounded theory, particularly interviews and observation, although literature review and relevant documentary analysis make important contributions. A key feature of grounded theory is the simultaneous collection and analysis of data using a process known as 'constant comparative analysis'. In this process, data are transcribed and examined for content immediately following data collection. Ideas which emerge from the analysis are included in data collection when the researcher next enters the field. For this reason, a researcher collecting data through semi-structured interviews may gradually develop an interview schedule in the latter stages of a research project which looks very different to the original schedule used in the first interview.

New theory begins its conception as the researcher recognises new ideas and themes emerging from what people have said or from events which have been observed. Memos form in the researcher's consciousness as raw data are reviewed. Hypotheses about the relationship between various ideas or categories are tested out and constructs formed, leading to new concepts or understandings. In this sense the theory is *grounded* in the data.

As in phenomenology, where there are concepts of which we are aware but do not fully understand, there are aspects of healthcare which might be informed by the development of new theory. One example is spirituality. In any holistic programme of care, healthcare professionals may talk about the need to meet the 'spiritual needs' of patients. However, we understand very little of what this means. At first sight, spiritual needs might be interpreted as referring to religious beliefs, but many people would say that spiritual needs are more than this. It may be an individual's sense of well-being, happiness or peace of mind. Grounded theory research could provide healthcare professionals with a better framework for providing truly holistic care.

Case study research

Like surveys, case study research is one of those research approaches which can take a qualitative or quantitative stance. In this chapter, the qualitative approach to case study is described wherein the value of case study relates to the in-depth analysis of a single or small number of units. Case study research is used to describe an entity that forms a single unit, such as a person, an organisation or an institution. Some research studies describe a series of cases.

Case study research ranges in complexity. The most simple is an illustrative description of a single event or occurrence. More complex is the analysis of a social situation over a period of time. The most complex is the extended case study which traces events involving the same actors over a period of time, enabling the analysis to reflect changes and adjustments.

As a research design, the case study claims to offer a richness and depth of information not usually offered by other methods. By attempting to capture as many variables as possible, case studies can identify how a complex set of circumstances come together to produce a particular manifestation. It is a highly versatile research method and employs any and all methods of data collection from testing to interviewing.

Case study research in healthcare has a range of uses. For example, a case study may be conducted into the development of a new service, such as a hospital discharge liaison scheme jointly run by health and social services in one locality. Another example of the case study approach would be to describe and analyse organisational change in the planning, purchasing or delivery of health services as in Total Purchasing pilot projects. One of the most common uses of the case study is the evaluation of a particular care approach. For example, an outreach teenage health service set up as an alternative to general practice-based teenage clinics might be evaluated in terms of input, impact on the health of teenagers locally, and the development of collaborative links with other groups involved in promoting teenage health.

One of the criticisms aimed at case study research is that the case under study is not necessarily representative of similar cases and therefore the results of the research are not generalisable. This is a misunderstanding of the purpose of case study research which is to describe *that particular case* in detail. It is particularistic and contextual. For example, the usefulness of an outreach teenage health service would be determined by a number of local factors and an evaluation of the service would take those factors into account. If the service works well, it does not automatically mean that the service would work equally well in another part of the country, but the lack of generalisability does not lessen the value of the service in the area where it is based. Generalisability is not normally an issue for the researcher who is involved in studying a specific situation. It is an issue for the readers who want to know whether the findings can be applied elsewhere. It is the readers who must decide whether or not the case being described is sufficiently representative or similar to their own local situation.

Summary

Four types of qualitative research design approaches have been outlined. They do not form an exhaustive list and some research methods can be applied with either a qualitative or a quantitative orientation. The language of qualitative research is not easy for the novice researcher to understand, as it often refers to abstract ideas, and this is not helped by diversity in the use of terms among qualitative writers.

The differences between the various qualitative research designs can be difficult to understand at first. The differences are quite subtle and are mainly concerned with the original research question, the people or situations being studied and the way the data are analysed, interpreted and presented. Readers should not worry if they do not fully understand the difference between phenomenology and grounded theory or between ethnography and case study at this stage in their reading. The main purpose of this section is to familiarise the reader with the notion that there are different qualitative methodologies and what the terms mean.

Exercise 2

Consider the following list of research problems and decide which would be the most appropriate qualitative research method for each one. If you think that more than one method would be appropriate, explain why.

1. The role of specialist nurses in community care.
2. Developing a primary healthcare service for the Chinese population in one city.
3. What is advocacy in primary healthcare?
4. An evaluation of the polyclinic – a one-stop primary healthcare centre.

Methods of collecting qualitative data

Qualitative approaches to data collection usually involve direct interaction with individuals on a one-to-one basis or in a group setting. Data collection methods are time-consuming and consequently data are collected from smaller numbers of people than would usually be the case in quantitative approaches, such as the questionnaire survey. The benefits of using these approaches include richness of data and deeper insight into the phenomena being studied.

Unlike quantitative data, raw qualitative data cannot be analysed statistically. The data from qualitative studies often derives from face-to-face interviews, focus groups or observation and so tends to be time-consuming to collect. Samples are usually smaller than with quantitative studies and are often locally based. Data analysis is also time-consuming and consequently expensive.

The main methods of collecting qualitative data are:

- individual interviews
- focus groups
- observation.

The interview

Interviews can be highly structured, semi-structured or unstructured. *Structured interviews* consist of the interviewer asking each respondent the same questions in the same way. A tightly structured schedule of questions is used, very much like a questionnaire. The questions may even be phrased in such a way that a limited range of responses can be elicited. For example: 'Do you think that health services in this area are excellent, good, average or poor?' Bearing in mind the cost of conducting a series of one-to-one interviews, the researcher planning to use structured interviews should carefully consider whether or not the information could be more efficiently collected using questionnaires.

Semi-structured interviews (sometimes referred to as focused interviews) involve a series of open-ended questions based on the topic areas the researcher wants to cover. The open-ended nature of the question defines the topic under investigation, but provides opportunities for both interviewer and interviewee to discuss some topics in more detail. If the interviewee has difficulty answering a question or provides only a brief response, the interviewer can use cues or prompts to encourage the interviewee to consider the question further. In a semi-structured interview the interviewer also has the freedom to probe the interviewee to elaborate on the original response or to follow a line of inquiry introduced by the interviewee. An example would be:

Interviewer: 'I'd like to hear your thoughts on whether changes in government policy have changed the work of the doctor in general practice. Has your work changed at all?'
Interviewee: 'Absolutely! The workload has increased for a start.'
Interviewer: 'In what way has it increased?'

Unstructured interviews (sometimes referred to as 'depth' or 'in-depth' interviews) have very little structure at all. The interviewer goes into the interview with the aim of discussing a limited number of topics, sometimes as few as one or two, and frames the questions on the basis of the interviewee's previous response. Although only one or two topics are discussed, they are covered in great detail. The interview might begin with the interviewer saying: 'I'd like to hear your views on GP commissioning'. Subsequent questions would depend on how the interviewee responded. Unstructured interviews are exactly what they sound like – interviews where the interviewer wants to find out about a specific topic but has no structure or preconceived plan or expectation as to how to deal with the topic. The difference with semi-structured interviews is that in a semi-structured interview the interviewer has a set of broad questions to ask and may also have some prompts to help the interviewee, but the interviewer has the time and space to respond to the interviewee's responses.

Qualitative interviews are semi-structured or unstructured. If the interview schedule is too tightly structured the phenomena under investigation may not be explored in terms of either breadth or depth. Semi-structured interviews tend to work well when the interviewer has already identified a number of aspects s/he wants to be sure of addressing. The interviewer can decide in advance what areas to cover, but is open and receptive to unexpected information from the interviewee. This can be particularly important if a limited time is available for each interview and the interviewer wants to be sure that the 'key issues' will be covered.

Qualitative interviews should be fairly informal. Interviewees should feel as though they are participating in a conversation or discussion rather than in a formal question-and-answer situation. However, achieving this informal style is dependent on careful planning and skill in conducting the interview. More information on the skills required of the interviewer can be found in Chapter 5 *Using interviews in a research project*.

Semi-structured interviews should not be seen as a soft option requiring little forethought. Good-quality qualitative interviews are the result of rigorous preparation. The development of the interview schedule, conducting the interview and analysing the interview data all require careful consideration and preparation. These matters are also discussed in Chapter 5 *Using interviews in a research project*.

Focus groups

Sometimes it is preferable to collect information from groups of people rather than from a series of individuals. Focus groups can be useful to obtain certain types of information, or when circumstances would make it difficult to collect information using other methods of data collection. They have been widely used in the private sector over the past few decades, particularly in market research, and are being used increasingly in the private sector. (See Chapter 5, *Using interviews in a research project*, for further details.)

Group interviews can be used when:

- limited resources prevent more than a small number of interviews to be undertaken
- it is possible to identify a number of individuals who share a common factor and it is desirable to collect the views of several people within that population subgroup
- group interaction among participants has the potential for greater insights to be developed.

Kreuger's *Focus Groups: A Practical Guide for Applied Research* (1994) provides comprehensive information on all aspects of focus groups. It is an excellent resource for anyone planning to use focus groups and contains further constructive advice that cannot be included in this volume due to the constraint of space.

Observation

Not all qualitative data collection approaches require direct interaction with people. Observation is a technique that can be used when data collected through other means are of limited value or difficult to validate. For example, in interviews, participants may be asked about how they behave in certain situations, but there is no guarantee that they actually do what they say they do. Observing them in those situations is more reliable: it is possible to see how they actually behave. Observation can also serve as a technique for verifying or nullifying information provided in face-to-face encounters.

In some research, it is not observation of people that is required but observation of the environment. This can provide valuable background information about the environment where a research project is being undertaken. For example, an action research project involving an institution may be enhanced by some description of the physical features of the building. An ethnographic study of an ethnic population may need information about how people dress or about their non-verbal communication. In a health-needs assessment, or in a locality survey, observations can provide broad descriptions of the key features of the area, e.g. whether the area is inner city, urban or rural, the geographical location, and the density of housing. It can describe the key components of the area: the main industries; type of housing. The availability of services can be identified: number, type and location of healthcare facilities such as hospitals and health centres; leisure facilities; and shopping centres.

Techniques for collecting data through observation

Written descriptions. The researcher can record observations of people, a situation or an environment by making notes of what has been observed. The limitations of this are similar to those of trying to write down interview data as it occurs. First there is a risk that the researcher will miss out on observations because s/he is writing about the last thing s/he noticed. Secondly, the researcher may find his/her attention focusing on a particular event or feature because they appear particularly interesting or relevant, and thus miss things which are equally or more important.

Video recording. This frees the observer from the task of making notes at the time and allows events to be reviewed time after time. One disadvantage of video recording is that the actors in the social world may be more conscious of the camera than they would be of a person and that their behaviour will be affected. They may even try to avoid being filmed. This problem can be lessened by having the camera placed in a fixed point rather than carried around. However, this means that only events in the line of the camera can be recorded, limiting the range of possible observations.

Photographs and artefacts. Photographs are a good way of collecting observable data of phenomena which can be captured in a single shot or series of shots. For example, photographs of buildings, neighbourhoods, dress and appearance. Artefacts are objects which inform us about the phenomenon under study because of their significance to the phenomena, for example memorabilia in historical research. Similarly, they may be instruments or tools used by members of a subgroup, whether this is a population subgroup or a professional or patient group.

Documentation. A wide range of written materials can produce qualitative information. They can be particularly useful in trying to understand the philosophy of an organisation as may be required in action research and case studies. They can include policy documents, mission statements, annual reports, minutes of meetings, codes of conduct, etc. Noticeboards can be a valuable source of data. Researchers who use this method of data collection sometimes develop a reputation as a 'lurker' because of their tendency to lurk around noticeboards!

More information about observation can be found in Chapter 6 *Data collection by observation*.

Handling qualitative research data

Interviewers have a choice of whether to take notes of responses during the interview or to tape-record the interview. The latter is preferable for a number of reasons. The interviewer can concentrate on listening and responding to the interviewee and is not distracted by trying to write down what has been said. The discussion flows because the interviewer does not have to write down the response to one question before moving on to the next. In note-taking there is an increased risk of interviewer bias because the interviewer is likely to make notes of the comments which make immediate sense or are perceived as being directly relevant or particularly interesting. Tape-recording ensures that the whole interview is captured and provides complete data for analysis so cues that were missed the first time can be recognised when listening to the recording. Lastly, interviewees may feel inhibited if the interviewer suddenly starts to scribble: they may wonder why what they have just said was of particular interest.

The ideal tape-recorder is small, unobtrusive and produces good-quality recording. An in-built microphone makes the participants less self-conscious. An auto-reverse facility is useful if the interview lasts longer than the recording time available on one side of the tape: this prevents an interruption in the flow of conversation. A tape-recorder with a counter facility can be useful when analysing the taped data (see below).

Transcribing qualitative data

Transcribing is the procedure for producing a written version of the interview. It is a full 'script' of the interview. Transcribing is a time-consuming process. The estimated ratio of time required for transcribing interviews is about 5:1. This means that it can take two and a half hours or more to transcribe a 30-minute interview. It also produces a lot of written text, as one interview can run to up to 20 pages.

The researcher should consider the question: Who should do the transcribing? If the research is funded or supported by an employer there may be resources to pay an audio typist. This is usually more cost-effective than a healthcare professional who will take longer and is more highly paid. However, if the transcriber is unfamiliar with the terminology or language contained in the interviews this can lead to mistakes or prolong the transcribing time.

Good-quality transcribing is not simply transferring words from the tape to the page. When people are in conversation only a small proportion of the message is communicated in the actual words used. A larger proportion is transmitted in the way people speak. Tone and inflection are good indicators of a whole range of feelings and meanings. When transcribing, consideration should be given to how these feelings and meanings can be communicated on paper by using punctuation marks and techniques such as upper-case lettering, underlining and emboldening. Take the phrase 'he was all right'. These four words can be said in a variety of ways and mean something different in every case.

'He was ALL RIGHT' (He was all right, I liked him)
'HE was all right' (He was all right, but I wasn't so keen on the others)
'He WAS all right' (He used to be all right, but he isn't now)
'He was all right?' (Well you might think so, but I don't)

By listening and noting the intensity and feeling in the interviewee's voice, it is possible to detect the following:

- positive/negative continuum: whether something was seen as good or bad
- certainty/uncertainty: how sure the interviewee was about what he said
- enthusiasm/reluctance: how happy or supportive the interviewee was about the topic being discussed.

It may not be essential to transcribe every interview. It is possible to use a technique known as 'tape analysis', which means taking notes from a playback of the tape-recorded interview. If tape analysis is used, the counter facility can be useful because the researcher can listen to the tape and make a note of the sections which contain particularly both useful information and key quotations, and return to these sections of the tape for fuller analysis. However, the previously mentioned problems of bias can occur if inexperienced qualitative researchers attempt tape analysis. It is certainly preferable to produce full transcripts of the first few interview data. Once the researcher becomes familiar with the key messages emerging from the data, tape analysis may be possible.

Another procedure sometimes adopted when interviews are used in qualitative research is 'constant comparative analysis'. This is a process whereby data collection and data analysis occur on an ongoing basis. The researcher conducts the first interview, which may be unstructured or semi-structured. The interview is transcribed and analysed as soon as possible, certainly before the next interview takes place, and any interesting findings are incorporated into the next interview. The process is repeated with each interview. When using this procedure it is quite possible that the initial interviews in a research project are very different to the later interviews, as the interview schedule has been continuously informed and revised by informants.

Analysing qualitative data

Analysis of data in a research project involves summarising the mass of data collected and presenting the results in a way that communicates the most important features. In quantitative research, analysis involves things like the frequencies of variables, differences between variables, statistical tests designed to estimate the significance of the results and the probability that they did not occur by chance. All this is done basically by counting how often something appears in the data and comparing one measurement with others. At the end of the analysis, not only do we have a mass of results, but we also have what we might call 'the big picture', the major findings.

In qualitative research we are also interested in discovering the big picture, but use different techniques to find it. As in quantitative research, there may be some data that are measurable but for the most part we are interested in using the data to describe a phenomenon, to articulate what it means and to understand it.

The basic process of analysing quantitative and qualitative data is the same. We start by labelling or coding every item of information so that we can recognise differences and similarities between all the different items. Imagine a questionnaire which has been used to collect quantitative information about why patients go to the health centre. The questionnaire might include a question like: Why did you last visit the health centre? Respondents have a choice of answers and tick the appropriate box. The researcher pre-codes the responses as follows:

I felt ill	= 1
To attend a health-screening clinic	= 2
To get a repeat prescription	= 3
A chiropody/physiotherapy appointment	= 4
I needed to get a form signed	= 5

The responses from all the questionnaires can be entered into a computer and the researcher can easily count up how many people answered the question in a given way – how many people went to the health centre because they felt ill, how many went to attend a health-screening clinic etc. Another question asks whether the respondent is male (coded as '1') or female (coded as '2'). Responses to this question can be considered in light of responses to the previous question by telling the computer to cross-tabulate responses. In this way it is possible to quickly tell, for example, how many men went to the doctor for health screening versus how many women.

Coding qualitative data requires different techniques. If, for example, the researcher has used a qualitative approach to explore patients' expectations of the health centre by

Qualitative research

interviewing patients, s/he will have a transcript of the interview with each patient, not a questionnaire. The researcher reads through the transcript and, at some point, finds reference to why the interviewee last visited the health centre. The qualitative researcher has no system for pre-coding, so needs a method of identifying and labelling (coding) items of data which appear in the text of a transcript so that all the items of data in one interview can be compared with data collected from other interviewees.

This requires a process called 'content analysis' and the basic procedure is described below. The procedure is the same whether the qualitative data has been collected through interviews, focus groups, observation or documentary analysis as it is concerned with analysing text.

Content analysis

Content analysis is a procedure for the categorisation of verbal or behavioural data, for purposes of classification, summarisation and tabulation. The content can be analysed on two levels. The basic level of analysis is a descriptive account of the data: this is what was actually said, with nothing read into it and nothing assumed about it. Some texts refer to this as the 'manifest level' or 'type of analysis'. The higher level of analysis is interpretative: it is concerned with what was meant by the response, what was inferred or implied. It is sometimes called the 'latent level of analysis'. Further information on content analysis can be found in Chapter 5 *Using interviews in a research project*.

Content analysis involves coding and classifying data. Some authors refer to this as 'categorising' or 'indexing'. The basic idea is to identify from the transcripts the extracts of data that are informative in some way and to sort out the important messages hidden in the mass of each interview.

The procedure involves a series of steps. These are listed as follows:

1. Take a copy of the transcript and read through it. When you see something that contains apparently interesting or relevant information, make a brief note in the margin about the nature of the information you have noticed.
2. Look through your margin notes and make a list of the different types of information you have found. If the transcript was typed using a word processor, a quicker way of doing this will be to highlight each item of data, copy it and paste it onto a list (make sure you keep an original copy of the whole transcript in your file!).
3. You now have a list of items excerpted from the text. Read through the list of data items and categorise each item in a way that describes what it is about. You will find yourself using some of the categories several times because several items of data refer to the same topic. However, at this stage go for as many categories as you need and don't put something into the same category as a previous item of data if you even suspect that you may have identified a new category. The number of categories can be reduced later.

4. Now look at the list of categories you have identified from the transcript and consider whether some of the categories may be linked in some way. If they can, you could list them as major categories and the original, smaller categories as minor categories. Some textbooks refer to these major categories as 'themes'.
5. Look through the list of minor and major categories of data. As you do so, compare and contrast the various categories. You may find that you change your mind about some of the minor categories. As you start to develop 'the big picture' you may perceive some items of data differently and see them as fitting better into an alternative category. Sometimes an item seems to belong in two categories. If so, list it under both.
6. Move on to the next transcript and repeat the process from stages 1–5. As you work through the second and subsequent transcripts you will continue to identify new categories of information, but you will increasingly find that you recognise an item of data as belonging to a previously identified category. Eventually you will run out of new categories and find that all the items of relevant and interesting information can be accommodated in the existing categories.

    At this stage some researchers like to colour-code their categories and use a different coloured highlighter pen for each category to highlight items of data in the transcripts. This is a good idea as it makes recognition of data easier when reviewing the transcripts at a later stage. However, be aware that you could change your mind later about an item of data and want to move it to a different category. Always keep clean copies of transcripts so that you can go over it with a different coloured pen.
7. Collect together all the extracts from the transcribed interviews that you have put into one category because they appeared to bear some relationship to each other. Examine each of the extracts in turn. Do they belong together or are there any extracts that now look as though they don't fit and really belong in a different category?
8. When all the relevant transcript data have been sorted into minor and major categories, look again at the data contained in each category. As you review the data within the system of categorisation you have developed you may decide to move some items of data from one category to another. Or you may decide that information is in the right category, in that it fits together, but the terms used to name or describe the category are inaccurate.
9. Once you have sorted out all the categories and are sure that all the items of data are in the right category, look at the range of categories to see whether two or more categories seem to fit together. If so they may form a major theme in your research.
10. Go back to the original copies of the transcripts, the ones where you made your initial notes in the margins. Look at any text that you did not highlight at all because it did not appear relevant at the time. Now you have the themes, and major and minor categories clearly sorted, consider whether any of the previously excluded data are relevant and should be included in your results.

Qualitative research

This process may appear confusing at first. It seems as though the qualitative researcher keeps changing his/her mind about data and has difficulty deciding what data belongs where. To some extent this is true. The process of content analysis involves continually revisiting the data and reviewing its categorisation until the researcher is sure that the themes and categories used to summarise and describe the findings are a truthful and accurate reflection of the data.

Exercise 3

It is not possible to demonstrate the complete procedure of content analysis within the space available for this chapter. However, this exercise provides an opportunity to look at an excerpt from a transcript and begin the process of categorising data.

The following text is an extract from the transcript of an interview conducted by a community psychiatric nurse with a woman following discharge from hospital. It deals with the woman's recollection of being admitted and how she felt at that time. Read the transcript carefully and complete the following tasks.

1. Make a note of all the items of data you consider to be potentially interesting.
2. Identify categories of data.
3. How many categories have you identified?
4. Do some items of data potentially relate to more than one category?
5. Can you identify major and minor categories?

Interviewer: What were your first impressions when you were first admitted to hospital?
Respondent: It's hard to remember. I was so terrified. I didn't know what to expect. I was so ashamed that I was going to a loony bin. I thought everybody would be mad. But then I saw Ann. I knew her and at first I couldn't believe it – she's not mad, why is she here? Then she came up to me and smiled and said hello and she started asking me about Bill and the kids. Then she asked me if I was visiting someone and I told her 'No, I've come in' and she told me why she was here. She didn't seem to think it was strange at all.
Interviewer: Who's Ann?
Respondent: She used to live next door to me at my last house before we moved.
Interviewer: So was it better when you saw Ann?
Respondent: Yes. Well, yes and no. It was good to see someone I knew but I didn't know what to think about it all. I mean, she was in there and I had no idea. Looking back a little while afterwards I realised that just because you go into a psychiatric hospital it doesn't mean you're mad. I wasn't and I knew she wasn't. Well, I hadn't thought so.
Interviewer: So before you arrived at the hospital, is that what you thought? That it would be full of mad people.
Respondent: Yes. Well you do don't you? But it wasn't. I was scared at first. But Ann stayed with me after the nurse had seen me and she talked to me about

	where we lived and everything and the people we knew and it was just like having a chat anywhere. It didn't feel like we were in hospital.
Interviewer:	How do you mean? Didn't the hospital look like you thought it would?
Respondent:	Not really. But looking back I don't know what picture I had of the hospital, only what the people would be like. And most of them were like you and me really. Only one or two seemed particularly ill. And I felt sorry for them. Only one chap I didn't like.
Interviewer:	Can I come back to that later? For now can we stick with your thoughts about your first impressions? I mean, for example, were the staff friendly? What about where you slept? The ward in general.
Respondent:	Well everyone was very kind. I think they knew I was frightened and they did their best to help. But they're busy. I'm glad Ann was there.
Interviewer:	What about the environment?
Respondent:	It was OK...ish. Not like a hospital. More like a lounge at a boarding house. A bit seedy. Needs decorating.
Interviewer:	How do you mean 'seedy'?
Respondent:	It needed decorating. And some of the chairs, you could fall through them if you weren't careful. I'm glad there was no smoking in the lounge but I think that had only started recently 'cos there were a lot of cigarette burns in the carpet. I don't like smoking. It makes me feel sick. Awful habit. The bedrooms were nice. They'd been decorated. And I loved the duvets and the curtains. You don't expect matching duvet and curtains. Mind you, one thing I didn't like about the bedrooms was that I couldn't lock my wardrobe...

Computerised data analysis

Software packages have been available for a long time to make analysis of quantitative data quicker and easier. In recent years software has been developed which can help with the analysis of qualitative data. An increasing range of packages is available, each one with different features, and some are more popular with new researchers than others. Essentially they work on the principle of recognising information and assisting with the process of categorisation, then collecting together items of information which appear to match under the given categories. The packages, if properly used, can save the researcher a great deal of time, but a fair amount of human input is still required to identify and check categorisation. They also require transcripts to be prepared on a computer, and some novices, particularly people conducting qualitative research as part of the coursework for a degree, may not have access to the IT resources necessary for computer analysis.

Some of the most well-known software packages are listed below.

- ATLAS/ti
- HyperRESEARCH

- Kwalitan
- QSR NUD*IST
- The Ethnograph v4.0

It is possible to access further information on many of these packages by looking on the Internet. Some companies have their own web sites. There are also a number of networks aimed at qualitative researchers which can be accessed via the Internet. One such network is CAQDAS, whose website address is http://www.soc.surrey.ac.uk/caqdas

Tape analysis

It is advisable, if at all possible, to analyse qualitative data using transcribed records of data. If transcripts of recorded interviews are not available it is possible to carry out tape analysis. This involves replaying the tape-recording of an interview and making notes of relevant and interesting data rather than full transcripts. It is much less time-consuming than transcript analysis, but it has a number of disadvantages. The procedure is open to researcher bias as the researcher is likely to make notes of information that is immediately recognisable as useful and potentially relevant information may be overlooked. The quality of the analysis may also lack depth and comprehensiveness. This can compromise the accuracy of data and therefore its reliability and validity.

Presenting the results of qualitative research

When planning the presentation of findings qualitative data have several features to take into consideration. The data are subjective, interpretative, descriptive, holistic and copious and it can be difficult to know where or how to start. A good starting point is to look at the themes and categories which have emerged and to use these to structure the results section of the research report.

This structure can be set out at the beginning, either as a list or in diagrammatic form. The themes are then presented in sections with the categories as subsections. In this way, the categories of data are used to construct a case that the themes are the main findings of the study. Further evidence to support the findings is provided by using direct quotations from respondents. Key quotations are selected to illustrate the meaning of the data. Consider Table 3.2, which shows the part of the structure of themes and categories which emerged from an investigation into the need for an outreach teenage health clinic.

A presentation of these findings would describe what was meant by 'health issues' in general for young people. This would be followed by identification and description of each of the broad categories of health issue – sexual health, drugs and mental health. Each category of health issue describes how a range of topics is included in this category (the minor categories). Quotations are extracted from the transcripts of interviews with young people to illustrate why or how this is a health issue.

Table 3.2

Themes	Major categories	Minor categories
1. Health issues for young people	sexual health	safe sex
		pregnancy
		sexual behaviour
		sexuality
	drugs	smoking
		alcohol
		illicit drugs
	mental health	mental health problems
		relationships
		self-esteem
		stress
2. Barriers to accessing services	lack of knowledge	services available
		understanding
		perceptions
	attitudes	own beliefs
		peer pressure
		expectations of staff
3. Incentives to use services	availability	time
		venue
	approachability	staff attributes
		environment

Quotations should be used because they are good examples of what people have said specifically about the category being described. A range of quotations should be selected to illustrate such features as: the strength of opinion or belief; similarities between respondents; differences between respondents; and the breadth of ideas.

As the researcher works through the different categories, links between categories should be made to demonstrate how the themes emerged and how conclusions about the findings were drawn. Many of the quotations will speak for themselves as they are examples of the manifest level of analysis – what people actually said. However, as previously mentioned, some analysis of data is carried out at the latent or interpretative level, which involves extracting the meaning of what was said. Careful selection of quotations will demonstrate the reliability and validity of the data analysis.

Some qualitative data can be dealt with in a quantitative way. If an idea appears in the data frequently it may be feasible to measure how often it appears. In the example of the teenage outreach service, it may be possible to say how many respondents identified sexual health as a health issue, how many identified drugs and how many identified mental health. By counting the number of respondents who mentioned contraception as opposed to the number who mentioned safe sex it may appear that contraception is a greater concern than safe sex for young people. It may be feasible or even desirable to present some of the results quantitatively using tables and figures. Using qualitative and quantitative techniques for analysis of data can strengthen the analysis.

Summary

The purpose of this chapter was to provide an introduction to qualitative research to enable readers with no previous knowledge to understand, at a basic level, how qualitative research is undertaken. By describing the nature of qualitative research and its different research designs, its potential to be used to investigate research problems in primary healthcare settings was demonstrated. Some of the issues involved in collecting and analysing qualitative data were addressed and the potential complexity of qualitative research was shown. This chapter is designed as a starting point for anyone contemplating qualitative research, but further reading is necessary to understand these complexities more fully. A selection of the more widely available texts is listed at the end of the chapter.

Answers to exercises

Exercise 1

1. Quantitative. In order for the effectiveness of the two drugs to be compared it would need to be *measured*.
2. Qualitative. The study aims to *explore* the role of the practice manager and will *describe a phenomenon*. The fact that the study is conducted in only four practices also suggests an *in-depth* study.
3. A *descriptive* study of *experience* suggests a qualitative approach. Also, the focus is boys with eating disorders and difficulty in locating a sizeable sample may be anticipated.
4. A *national survey* suggests a *large-scale* study. The data could be collected using a *questionnaire*.

Exercise 2

1. Phenomenology – the study seeks to explore and describe a phenomena.
2. Ethnography – to inform the development of a service for a particular cultural group, the research would seek to understand the beliefs and practices of the culture.
3. Grounded theory – if we can understand and describe what advocacy actually *means* in primary healthcare, the new knowledge can be incorporated into practices and policy.
4. Case study – the polyclinic is a 'case', a unit of study.

Exercise 3

1. At this stage, all the information is new and everything is potentially interesting.
2. You are likely to have identified some or all of the following categories:
   - feelings of the respondent – fear, embarrassment or shame, surprise

- beliefs about people with mental illness – who they are and how they appear
- expectations of the hospital
- attitude towards smoking
- concerns about security.

3. Your categorisation may be broader or narrower than this; consequently the numbers of categories may be different. But isn't it interesting that so many categories can be generated from one page of transcript?
4. As an example, expectations and beliefs might be one or two categories.
5. For example, feelings of the respondent might be a major category and the different feelings could be minor categories. You would decide as further interview transcripts were analysed.

References and further reading

Bryman A and Burgess R (eds) (1993) *Analysing Qualitative Data*. Routledge, London.

Burnard P (1991) A method of analysing interview transcripts in qualitative research. *Nurse Education Today*. **11**: 461–66.

Burnard P (1994) Using a database programme to handle qualitative data. *Nurse Education Today*. **14**(3): 228–31.

Carter Y and Thomas C (eds) (1997) *Research Methods in Primary Care*. Radcliffe Medical Press, Oxford.

Cobb A K and Hagemaster J N (1987) Ten criteria for evaluating qualitative research proposals. *Journal of Nursing Education*. **26**(4): 138–43.

Cooke M (1992) Computer analyses of qualitative data: a literature review of current issues. *Australian Journal of Advanced Nursing*. **10**(1): 10–13.

Glaser B G and Strauss A L (1967) *The Discovery of Grounded Theory*. Aldine, Chicago.

Hammersley M and Atkinson P (1989) *Ethnography: Principles in Practice*. Routledge, London.

Kreuger R A (1994) *Focus Groups: A Practical Guide For Applied Research* (2e). Sage, London.

Leininger M M (1985) *Qualitative Research Methods in Nursing*. Harcourt Brace & Co, London.

Maykut P and Morehouse R (1994) *Beginning Qualitative Research: A Philosophical and Practical Guide*. Falmer, London.

Mays N and Pope C (eds) (1996) *Qualitative Research in Health Care*. BMJ Publishing Group, London.

Miles M and Huberman A (1994) *Qualitative Data Analysis*. Sage, Thousand Oaks.

Silverman D (1993) *Interpreting Qualitative Data: Methods For Analysing Talk, Text and Interaction*. Sage, London.

Sorrell J M and Redmond G M (1995) Interviews in qualitative nursing research: differing approaches for ethnographic and phenomenological studies. *Journal of Advance Nursing*. **21**(6): 1117–22.

Stake R E (1995) *The Art of Case Study Research*. Sage, Thousand Oaks.

Strauss A and Corbin J (1990) *Basics of Qualitative Research: Grounded Theory Procedures and Techniques*. Sage, London.

Yin R K (1994) *Case Study Research: Design and Methods* (2e). Sage, Newbury Park.

CHAPTER FOUR

Surveys and questionnaires

Nigel Mathers, Nick Fox and Amanda Hunn

Introduction

The survey is probably the most commonly used research design in health services research and the social sciences. We have all been asked to take part in a survey at some time. As consumers we are asked about our shopping habits, as users of services we are asked for our opinions of services.

The survey is a flexible research approach used to investigate a wide range of topics. Surveys often employ the questionnaire as a tool for data collection. This chapter considers the use of surveys and questionnaires in primary healthcare research.

Having successfully completed the work in this chapter, you will be able to:

- understand why you might want to use a survey
- describe how to select a sample for a survey
- understand why you might want to use a questionnaire
- understand how the method used for data collection influences the design of the questionnaire
- distinguish between a structured questionnaire, semi-structured questionnaire and a topic guide
- design your own questionnaire and coding frame
- distinguish between open-ended and closed questions
- list possible ways of increasing your response rate.

What is a survey?

Surveys are a very traditional way of conducting research. They are particularly useful for non-experimental descriptive designs that seek to describe reality. So, for instance, a survey approach may be used to establish the prevalence or incidence of a particular condition. Likewise, the survey approach is frequently used to collect information on attitudes and behaviour. This means that surveys are a useful and practical approach to take when conducting research in a primary care setting. Some issues are best addressed by classical experimental design where subjects are randomised to either an intervention group or a control group. In the real world it is not always a very practical design. There may be good reasons, either ethical or practical, why subjects cannot be randomly assigned to a particular intervention. It may also be impossible to identify a control group. Surveys are often a very acceptable alternative approach. Whilst it is perfectly possible to use experimental designs in a primary care setting, it can often be very complex to set up and manage, particularly when the subjects have to be recruited across a very large number of general practices. Control over the randomisation process can be difficult to achieve. It is much easier to set up a study with an experimental approach in a hospital setting where patients with a particular condition can be easily identified and randomised into intervention and control groups.

Surveys can take many forms. A survey of the entire population would be known as a census. However, surveys are usually restricted to a representative sample of the potential group that the researcher is interested in, for reasons of practicality and cost-effectiveness. Most surveys take one of the following forms:

Cross-sectional surveys

Surveys that are carried out at just one point in time are known as cross-sectional in design. They provide us with a snapshot of what is happening at that particular time. They usually take a descriptive or exploratory form that simply sets out to describe behaviour or attitudes. So for example, if you want to measure some aspect of patient satisfaction amongst your patients, then a cross-sectional descriptive survey would be the recommended approach. Likewise, if you wish to establish the prevalence of urinary incontinence amongst new mothers, a postal survey might be an appropriate approach.

Longitudinal surveys

Alternatively surveys can be longitudinal. A longitudinal survey, rather than taking a snapshot, paints a picture of events or attitudes over time. This may be a matter of months or years. There may be only two discrete surveys or there may be many repeated waves over a long period of time. Longitudinal surveys usually take one of two forms:

- cohort surveys – which follow the same group of individuals over time
- trend surveys – which take repeated samples of different people each time, but always use the same core questions.

Cohort studies are particularly useful in tracking the progress of particular conditions over time, whereas trend studies set out to measure trends in public opinion and behaviour over time. For instance, take the patient satisfaction survey which was mentioned earlier. If we wanted to compare levels of patient satisfaction year on year, then a longitudinal trend survey would be recommended. With a trend study it is not necessary to interview the same individuals each time. In fact it is probably better to deliberately avoid the same people since the very fact of participating in a survey can raise levels of awareness and change behaviour. This is particularly true if you are trying to measure awareness of a health promotion campaign. A particularly well-known version of a trend survey is the General Household Survey, which is carried out on an annual basis.

A cohort study is more difficult to carry out than a trend survey because the same individuals have to be traced over time and inevitably some subjects move house, some fall ill and die, and some just refuse to participate. This loss of subjects is known as 'attrition'. Sample size calculations are even more important for cohort surveys because high levels of attrition can result in too small a sample in the final stages of the survey. Ideally, expected levels of attrition should be calculated and allowed for in the initial sample selection. This means that the early stages of the cohort may be unnecessarily large but in turn this means that you will have adequate numbers in the final wave. A fine example of a cohort study is the National Child Development Study, which is based on an initial sample of children born in one week in 1947 and continued to follow them through over many years.

Explanatory or correlational surveys

We have described how some surveys seek only to describe events and attitudes. It is also possible for surveys to take an explanatory or correlational approach. This means that by using survey data the researcher would try to explore causal relationships between two or more variables. Demonstrating a causal relationship using survey data will always be more difficult than using an experimental design. Nevertheless there will always be situations in which an experimental design is just not possible. Using a longitudinal approach may also help in trying to identify a causal relationship. Statistical tests can be used to show statistically significant differences between groups in a survey. Confounding variables can also be controlled for in the data analysis.

Advantages of using a survey

Internal and external validity

A survey which is based on some form of random sampling technique will produce a sample which is representative of the particular population under study and findings which may be generalised to the wider population. Randomised clinical trials (RCTs), on the other hand, often have very stringent inclusion and exclusion criteria which make generalisations of the findings very difficult to apply in the real world.

Efficiency

Because surveys can use a random sampling technique to recruit subjects, relatively small sample sizes can be used to generate findings which can be used to draw conclusions about the whole population. They are thus a very cost-effective way of finding out what people do, think and want.

Cover geographically spread samples
Surveys can be undertaken using a wide range of techniques, including postal questionnaires and telephone interviews. This means that subjects who are widely dispersed can be accessed and included in the sample.

Ethical advantages
Since most surveys do not expose individuals to possibly invasive techniques or withhold treatment, they may be considered more ethical, since the individuals included in a study will merely be exposed to events that occur in the real world and would have taken place anyway.

Flexibility
Surveys can easily be combined with other methods to produce richer data. So, for instance, you might want to consider also using symptom diaries, focus groups, or in-depth interviews.

Limitations of using a survey

Dependency upon the chosen sampling frame
The representativeness of a survey is entirely dependent upon the accuracy of the sampling frame used. Sometimes it is not possible to identify an accurate or up-to-date sampling frame.

Inability to explain why people think or act as they do
Surveys can tell us how many people behave in a certain way or how many patients were dissatisfied with their treatment, but they may be limited in the information they can provide as to *why* this is so (although asking open-ended questions can allow you to find out more). Qualitative research is usually much better at answering 'why' questions.

Interview surveys are only as good as the interviewers asking the questions
The outcome of a survey may be influenced by interviewer error and bias. It is important that all interviewers receive proper training and are thoroughly briefed on each project.

Methods of collecting survey data

It is important to remember that a survey is a type of research design. In contrast, an interview or a postal questionnaire is a method of data collection. There is a wide range of methods available for collecting data covering human subjects, but the three main methods of collecting survey data are:

- face-to-face interviews
- telephone interviews
- questionnaires.

The selection of the appropriate method depends upon a number of factors, including:

- access to potential subjects/respondents
- the literacy level of respondents
- the subject matter
- the motivation of the respondents
- resources.

We will now cover each method in more detail.

Face-to-face surveys

Face-to-face or personal interviews are very labour intensive, but can be the best way of collecting high-quality data. Face-to-face interviews are preferable:

- when the subject matter is very sensitive
- if the questions to be coded are very complex
- if the interview is likely to be lengthy.

Face-to-face interviews can take both qualitative and quantitative approaches, but surveys tend to take a quantitative approach. Interviewers carrying out face-to-face interviews for a quantitative study will use a highly structured interview schedule. Overall face-to-face interviews are more expensive and costly than other methods, but they can collect more complex information and are also useful when the subject matter is not of great personal interest to the respondent and who would therefore be unlikely to complete a postal questionnaire.

Telephone surveys

Telephone interviews can be a very effective and economical way of collecting quantitative data, if the individuals in the sampling frame can all equally be accessed via a telephone and if the questionnaire is fairly short. This may not be an appropriate method for a deprived population where telephone ownership is likely to be low, but can be ideally suited to a busy professional respondent, such as a general practitioner or a hospital consultant, if prior appointments are made. Telephone interviews are particularly useful when the respondents to be interviewed are geographically widely distributed. However, the complexity of the interview is limited without the use of visual aids and prompts. The length of a telephone interview is also limited, although this will vary with subject area and motivation. A prior appointment and covering letter may enhance the response rate and length of interview.

When it comes to data collection, telephone interviews are sometimes recorded using a tape-recorder or the answers can be typed directly into a computer as the interview is being conducted.

When doing a face-to-face or telephone survey of respondents in their own homes it is important to do some evening calling, otherwise the survey may be restricted to those who are at home during the day. For guidelines on conducting a face-to-face or telephone interview see Chapter 5 *Using interviews in a research project*.

Questionnaires

Questionnaires are a useful option to consider when conducting a postal survey. They are cheaper than personal interviewing and quicker if the sample is large and widely dispersed. For any postal survey, regardless of the sample size, you must allow at least six weeks for the first wave of questionnaires to be returned, and another four weeks for each successive mailing. As with telephone interviewing, a postal survey is useful if your respondents are widely distributed. However, due to the lack of personal contact between the respondent and the researcher, the design and layout of the questionnaire is all-important.

All mailed questionnaires should be accompanied by a covering letter. In general, postal surveys tend to have lower response rates than face-to-face interviews. However, questionnaires sent to patient populations with a covering letter from their general practitioner tend to have very high response rates. Conversely postal surveys of general practitioners tend to produce low response rates.

As an alternative to mailing the questionnaire, it is possible to hand them out directly to your potential respondents in your chosen sampling frame. For instance you may decide that questionnaires can be handed out directly to parents with young children attending the surgery for a consultation. Another example might be a health visitor visiting mothers six weeks after birth and asking them to complete a questionnaire. In both cases it is relatively easy to approach respondents in these circumstances and you are likely to achieve a much higher response rate than would be possible with a postal survey. The main drawback of this approach is that your captive audience may in some way be biased. For example, if you carry out a survey of patient satisfaction which is restricted only to those patients attending in surgery, then the results will be biased towards the views of the most frequent attenders and consequently those people with most health problems.

Questionnaires can either be devised by the researcher or based upon some ready-made index such as the SF36 or GHQ. If you choose to design your own questionnaire for self-completion, then the rules governing the style and layout are the same as those for designing a questionnaire for a postal survey.

There are now many pre-existing questionnaires covering a wide range of conditions and therapy areas as well as quality of life instruments and patient satisfaction measures. Some of these are designed for self-completion, others are designed to be administered by an interviewer. There are obvious advantages of using such questionnaires, including the fact that many of these have already been well validated and tested for reliability, and there may well be normative data available as a baseline against which to compare your results. You need to be careful, however, that the questionnaire of choice was not designed firstly, with another culture in mind, and secondly, for use in secondary care settings only. Many questionnaires have been adapted to individual countries and also to the primary care setting, but you need to check first.

Remember there is no need to reinvent the wheel, so before designing your own questionnaire, you should spend time investigating what material exists already (see Box 4.1).

Many of these questionnaires are copyright protected and you may need the author's permission to use them. Likewise, using some questionnaires incurs a charge for each subject. You will therefore need to check whether or not there is a charge before you decide which questionnaire to use.

Box 4.1   Examples of existing health outcome measures or indices

- the **GHQ** – the General Health Questionnaire, which is designed to detect non-psychotic psychiatric illness in a community setting
- the **Short Form** (SF) 20 or 36 item Health Survey, which is a general health survey measure used to measure health status, both physical and mental
- the **Functional Limitations Profile** (FLP) for measuring the impact of illness on functioning

For details of these and other instruments, contact: the UK Clearing House on Health Outcomes at the Nuffield Institute for Health, 71–75 Clarendon Road, Leeds LS2 9PL. Tel: 0113 233 3940; Fax: 0113 246 0899; E-mail: hsschho@leeds.ac.uk.

Exercise 1

1. What are the three most important advantages of a face-to-face interview survey?
2. What are the three main disadvantages of a face-to-face interview survey?

Exercise 2
1. What are the main advantages of a telephone survey?
2. What are the main disadvantages of a telephone survey?

Exercise 3
1. What are the main advantages of a postal survey?
2. What the main disadvantages of a postal survey?

Sampling for surveys

Why do we need to select a sample?

In some instances the sample for your study may be the same as the population under investigation. If the subjects of your study are very rare, for instance a disease occurring only once in 100 000 children, then you might decide to study every case you can find. More usually, however, you are likely to find yourself in a situation where the potential subjects of your study are much more common and you cannot practically include everybody.

So it is necessary to find some way of reducing the number of subjects included in the survey without biasing the findings in any way. Random sampling is one way of achieving this, and with appropriate statistics such a study can yield valid findings at far lower cost. Samples can also be taken using non-random techniques, but in this chapter we will emphasise random sampling, which – if conducted adequately – will ensure internal validity.

Random sampling

To obtain a random (or probability) sample, the first step is to define the population from which it is to be drawn. This population is known as the *sampling frame*. For instance, you are interested in doing a survey of children aged between two and ten years diagnosed within the last month as having otitis media. Or you want to study adults (aged 16–65 years) diagnosed as having asthma and receiving drug treatment for asthma in the last six months, and living in a defined geographical region. In each case, these limits define the sampling frame.

The term *random* may imply to you that it is possible to take some sort of haphazard or *ad hoc* approach, for example stopping the first 20 people you meet in the street for inclusion in your study. This is not random in the true sense of the word. To be a random sample, every individual in the population must have an equal probability of being selected. In order to carry out random sampling properly, strict procedures need to be adhered to.

Random sampling techniques can be split into *simple random sampling* and *systematic random sampling*.

Simple random sampling

If selections are made purely by chance this is known as simple random sampling. So, for instance, if we had a population containing 5000 people, we could allocate every individual a different number. If we wanted to achieve a sample size of 200, we could achieve this by pulling 200 of the 5000 numbers out of a hat. Another way of selecting the numbers would be to use a table of random numbers. These tables are usually to be found in the appendices of most statistical textbooks.

Systematic random sampling

Systematic random sampling is a more commonly employed method. After numbers are allocated to everybody in the population frame, the first individual is picked using a random number table and then subsequent subjects are selected using a fixed sampling interval, i.e. every *nth* person.

Assume, for example, that we wanted to carry out a survey of patients with asthma attending clinics in one city. There may be too many to interview everyone, so we want to select a representative sample. If there are 3000 people attending the clinics in total and we only require a sample of 200, we would need to:

- calculate the sampling interval by dividing 3000 by 200 to give a sampling fraction of 15
- select a random number between one and 15 using a set of random tables
- if this number were 13, we select the individual allocated number 13 and then go on to select every 15th person.

This will give us a total sample size of 200 as required.

Care needs to be taken when using a systematic random sampling method in case there is some bias in the way that lists of individuals are compiled, for example if all the husbands' names precede wives' names and the sampling interval is an even number, then we may end up selecting all women and no men.

Stratified random sampling

Stratified random sampling is a way of ensuring that particular strata or categories of individuals are represented in the sampling process.

If, for example, we want to study consultation rates in a general practice, and we know that approximately 4% of our population frame is made up of a particular ethnic minority group, there is a chance that with simple or systematic random sampling we could end up with no ethnic minorities (or a much-reduced proportion) in our sample. If we wanted to ensure that our sample was representative of the population frame, then we would employ a stratified sampling method as follows:

1. First we would split the population into the different strata, in this case, separating out those individuals with the relevant ethnic background.
2. We would then apply random sampling techniques to each of the two ethnic groups separately, using the same sampling interval in each group.
3. This would ensure that the final sampling frame was representative of the minority group we wanted to include, on a pro rata basis with the actual population.

Disproportionate sampling

Taking this example once more, if our objective was to compare the results of our minority group with the larger group, then we would have difficulty in doing so, using the proportionate stratified sampling just described, because the numbers achieved in the minority group, although pro rata those of the population, would not be large enough to demonstrate statistical differences.

To compare the survey results of the minority individuals with those of the larger group, it is necessary to use a disproportionate sampling method. With disproportionate sampling, the strata are not selected pro rata to their size in the wider population. For instance, if we are interested in comparing the referral rates for particular minority groups with other larger groups, then it is necessary to over-sample the smaller categories in order to achieve statistical power, that is, in order to be able to demonstrate statistically significant differences between groups.

(Note that if subsequently we wish to refer to the total sample as a whole, representative of the wider population, then it will become necessary to re-weight the categories back into the proportions in which they are represented in reality. For example, if we wanted to compare the views and satisfaction levels of women who gave birth at home compared with the majority of women who gave birth in hospital, a systematic random sample, although representative of all women giving birth, would not produce a sufficient number of women giving birth at home to be able to compare the results, unless the total sample was so big that it would take many years to collate. We would also end up interviewing more women than we needed who have given birth in hospital. In this case it would be necessary to over-sample or over-represent those women giving birth at home to have enough individuals in each group in order to compare them. We would therefore use disproportionate stratified random sampling to select the sample.)

The important thing to note here about disproportionate sampling is that randomisation is still taking place within each stratum or category. So we would use systematic random selection to select a sample from the majority group and the same process to select samples from the minority groups.

Cluster sampling

Cluster sampling is a method frequently employed in national surveys where it is uneconomic to carry out interviews with individuals scattered across the country. Cluster

Surveys and questionnaires

sampling allows individuals to be selected in geographical batches. So, for instance, before selecting at random, the researcher may decide to focus on certain towns, electoral wards or general practices. Multi-stage sampling allows the individuals within the selected cluster units to then be selected at random.

Obviously care must be taken to ensure that the cluster units selected are generally representative of the population and are not strongly biased in any way. If, for example, all the general practices selected for a study were fundholding, this would not be representative of all general practice.

Note that even if the researcher randomly selects the initial clusters this does not constitute a truly random sampling method.

Non-random sampling

Non-random (or non-probability) sampling is not used very often in quantitative social research, but it is increasingly used in market research surveys and commissioned studies. The technique most commonly used is known as quota sampling.

Quota sampling

Quota sampling is a technique whereby the researcher decides in advance on certain key characteristics which s/he will use to stratify the sample. Interviewers are often set sample quotas in terms of age and sex. So, for example, with a sample of 200 people, they may decide that 50% should be male and 50% should be female; and 40% should be aged over 40 years and 60% aged 39 years or less. The difference with a stratified sample is that the respondents in a quota sample are not randomly selected within the strata. The respondents may be selected just because they are accessible to the interviewer. Because random sampling is not employed, it is not possible to apply inferential statistics and generalise the findings to a wider population.

Convenience or opportunistic sampling

Selecting respondents purely because they are easily accessible is known as convenience sampling. Whilst this technique is generally frowned upon by quantitative researchers, it is regarded as an acceptable approach when using a qualitative design, since generalisability is not a main aim of qualitative approaches.

Exercise 4

Read the descriptions below and decide what type of sample selection has taken place.

1. Schoolchildren, some with asthma and some without, are identified from GP records. Method: children are selected randomly within each of the two groups and the number of children in each group is representative of the total patient population for this age group.

2. Children with and without chronic asthma are identified from GP records. Method: the children are selected so that exactly 50% have chronic asthma and 50% have no asthma. Within each group, the children are randomly selected.
3. A survey of the attitudes of mothers with children under one year. Method: interviewers stop likely-looking women pushing prams in the street. The number of respondents who fall into different age bands and social classes is strictly controlled.
4. A survey of attitudes of drug users to rehabilitation services. Method: drug users are recruited by advertising in the local newspaper for potential respondents.
5. A postal survey of the attitudes of males to use of male contraceptives. Method: all male adults whose national insurance numbers end in '5' are selected for a survey.
6. A study of the length of stay of patients at Anytown General Hospital. Method: all patients admitted to wards 3, 5, and 10 in a hospital are selected for a study.

Exercise 5

This is an opportunity to review your learning from the first part of this chapter. Read the extract from a journal article 'National asthma survey reveals continuing morbidity' below.

National asthma survey reveals continuing morbidity
(*Prescriber*, 19 March 1996)

'A preliminary analysis of a survey of 44,177 people with asthma has revealed that for many the condition causes frequent symptoms and substantially interferes with daily life. There is also a trend for older people with asthma to experience more problems. More information about treatment was seen by many as the best way to improve care.

The Impact of Asthma Survey was conducted by Gallup on behalf of the National Asthma Campaign with funding from Allen & Hanburys. Questionnaires were given to people with asthma via surgeries, pharmacies, retail outlets, the media and direct mailing in the autumn of 1995; the respondents were therefore self-selected and may not be representative of the population with asthma.

Asthma symptoms were experienced on most days or daily by 41% of survey respondents, ranging from 18% of the under-11s to 55% of pensioners. Waking every night with wheeze, cough or breathlessness was reported by 13% and 43% say they are woken by symptoms at least once a week.

About 20% consider that asthma dominates their life, ranging from 17% in children to 37% in the over-60s; over 40% of each age group say the condition has a moderate impact on their quality of life.'

Now answer the following questions.

1. How was the sample selected for this survey?
2. Did the researchers use random or non-random sampling methods?
3. What are the advantages of their approach?
4. What are the disadvantages of this approach?

5. The sample size was 44 177. Why was the sample size so large and was this necessary?

Sample size

For details on how to calculate the required sample size you should refer to the Trent Focus research volume *Statistical Analysis in Primary Care*, Chapter 2 'Sampling'. Bear in mind that if you intend to carry out a survey to calculate a proportion or a mean figure, you will need to consider the width of the confidence interval around the figure you produce. The confidence interval is the margin of error that surrounds your result. No survey can produce a result that is precisely correct. By sampling, we are aiming to achieve a degree of acceptable accuracy. There is likely to be a margin of error around any figure that you produce as a result of a survey. For example, if we survey 300 patients randomly selected from a general practitioner's records and find that 75% say that they were satisfied with the care they received at their last consultation, we can be 95% certain that the true answer is 5% either side of 75% (i.e. between 70% and 80%). This is known as the 95% confidence interval.

Table 4.1 can be used to calculate the required sample size for your survey given any particular percentage response. For example, if we plan to repeat the above survey and know that last time we had a response rate of 75%, we find the figure of 75% in the band at the top of the table and we then move down the table column until we find an acceptable margin of error in that column and an acceptable sample size in the left-hand column.

If we decide that a margin of error of 5% either way is too great and we need a greater level of accuracy, e.g. 2%, then we move down the column headed 75% until we hit 2% (1.9% is the nearest figure). In the left-hand column we can see that we will need a sample size of 2000 to achieve this.

Remember also that you will need to allow for the expected non-response to your survey and add this to your initial sample size. For instance, if you guess that only 50% of your sample will respond to your survey, then you will need to double your required sample size.

If in doubt about what percentage figure to expect in your results, then assume the outcome to be 50%. This is represented by the far right-hand column of the table and gives the worst-case scenario for estimating sample size. So, for instance, if we want to find out what percentage of patients self-treat with medicines they purchase themselves before visiting the doctor with a URTI and we cannot guess the answer, we should assume it is 50% for the purpose of calculating the sample size for our survey. Assuming that we want a very precise answer which is plus or minus 2%, then using the far right-hand column of the table shows that we will require a sample size of 2500.

Use this table if you want to be 'reasonably sure' (20–1 odds – i.e. at 95% confidence interval) of not exceeding the range of error.

Table 4.1

	PERCENTAGE OF RESPONDENTS GIVING A CERTAIN ANSWER

Sample size	1% or 99%	2% or 98%	3% or 97%	4% or 96%	5% or 95%	6% or 94%	8% or 92%	10% or 90%	12% or 88%	15% or 85%	20% or 80%	25% or 75%	30% or 70%	35% or 65%	40% or 60%	45% or 55%

	RANGE OF ERROR (PERCENTAGE PLUS OR MINUS) IS SHOWN BELOW

Sample size																
25	4.0	5.6	6.8	7.8	8.7	9.5	10.8	12.0	13.0	14.3	16.0	17.3	18.3	19.1	19.6	19.8
50	2.8	4.0	4.9	5.6	6.2	6.8	7.7	8.5	9.2	10.1	11.4	12.3	13.0	13.5	13.9	14.1
75	2.3	3.2	3.9	4.5	5.0	5.5	6.2	6.9	7.5	8.2	9.2	10.0	10.5	11.0	11.3	11.4
100	2.0	2.8	3.4	3.9	4.4	4.8	5.4	6.0	6.5	7.1	8.0	8.7	9.2	9.5	9.8	9.9
150	1.6	2.3	2.8	3.2	3.6	3.9	4.4	4.9	5.3	5.9	6.6	7.1	7.5	7.8	8.0	8.1
200	1.4	2.0	2.4	2.8	3.1	3.4	3.8	4.3	4.6	5.1	5.7	6.1	6.5	6.8	7.0	7.0
250	1.2	1.8	2.2	2.5	2.7	3.0	3.4	3.8	4.1	4.5	5.0	5.5	5.8	6.0	6.2	6.2
300	1.1	1.6	2.0	2.3	2.5	2.8	3.1	3.5	3.8	4.1	4.6	5.0	5.3	5.5	5.7	5.8
400	.99	1.4	1.7	2.0	2.2	2.4	2.7	3.0	3.3	3.6	4.0	4.3	4.6	4.8	4.9	5.0
500	.89	1.3	1.5	1.8	2.0	2.1	2.4	2.7	2.9	3.2	3.6	3.9	4.1	4.3	4.4	4.5
600	.81	1.1	1.4	1.6	1.8	2.0	2.2	2.5	2.7	2.9	3.3	3.6	3.8	3.8	4.0	4.1
800	.69	.98	1.2	1.4	1.5	1.7	1.9	2.1	2.3	2.5	2.8	3.0	3.2	3.3	3.4	3.5
1000	.63	.90	1.1	1.3	1.4	1.5	1.7	1.9	2.1	2.3	2.6	2.8	2.9	3.1	3.1	3.2
1200	.57	.81	.99	1.1	1.3	1.4	1.6	1.7	1.9	2.1	2.3	2.5	2.7	2.8	2.8	2.9
1500	.51	.73	.89	1.0	1.1	1.2	1.4	1.6	1.7	1.9	2.1	2.3	2.4	2.5	2.5	2.6
2000	.44	.61	.75	.86	.96	1.0	1.2	1.3	1.4	1.6	1.8	1.9	2.0	2.1	2.2	2.2
2500	.40	.56	.68	.78	.87	.95	1.1	1.2	1.3	1.4	1.6	1.7	1.8	1.9	2.0	2.0
3000	.36	.51	.62	.71	.79	.87	.99	1.1	1.2	1.3	1.5	1.6	1.7	1.7	1.8	1.8
4000	.31	.44	.54	.62	.69	.75	.86	.95	1.0	1.1	1.3	1.4	1.4	1.5	1.5	1.6
5000	.28	.40	.49	.56	.62	.68	.77	.85	.92	1.0	1.1	1.2	1.3	1.4	1.4	1.4
7500	.23	.32	.39	.45	.50	.55	.62	.69	.75	.82	.92	1.0	1.1	1.1	1.1	1.1
10000	.20	.28	.34	.39	.44	.48	.54	.60	.65	.71	.80	.87	.92	.95	.98	.99
15000	.16	.23	.28	.32	.36	.39	.44	.49	.53	.59	.66	.71	.75	.78	.80	.81
25000	.12	.18	.22	.25	.27	.30	.34	.38	.41	.45	.50	.55	.58	.56	.62	.62
50000	.08	.11	.14	.16	.17	.19	.22	.24	.26	.29	.32	.35	.39	.39	.39	.40

Questionnaire design

Questionnaires are a very convenient way of collecting useful comparable data from a large number of individuals. However questionnaires can only produce valid and meaningful results if the questions are clear and precise and if they are asked consistently across all respondents. Careful consideration therefore needs to be given to the design of the questionnaire.

All questionnaires should take into account:

1. Whether the questionnaire will be self-completion. Questionnaires can be administered face-to-face by an interviewer, by the telephone or completed independently by the subjects. The distinction between these methods is important because it has profound effects on the questionnaire design. A questionnaire which is to be completed by the respondent needs to be very clearly laid out, with no complex filtering, and simple instructions. Whereas a questionnaire to be administered by an interviewer can be much more complex.
2. The literacy level of the respondents. Obviously respondents with low literacy levels will have greater difficulty completing a self-completion or postal questionnaire. In this case a face-to-face or telephone interview survey would be advisable.
3. The expected response rate. The more motivated the respondent, the more likely you are to get a questionnaire returned in a postal survey. If you anticipate a very good response rate then a postal survey may do. If, on the other hand, you expect a low response rate, then a personal interview survey is likely to achieve higher acquiescence.
4. The resources available. One person would take a very long time to interview 1000 people, however one person could carry out a postal survey of the same number of respondents with relative ease.
5. Topic and population of interest. Finally it is important to bear in mind that you do not need to reinvent the wheel. Increasingly there are ready-made questionnaires and scales available to measure patient need and outcome. Many of these are commonly used, have been well validated and can also offer useful normative data for comparison. These will be discussed in more detail later in the chapter.

The title

All questionnaires require a title. It needs to be appealing and inviting, not the full academic title of the study.

The identifier

Each questionnaire will also probably require a subject identifier. If your survey is confidential, i.e. you know the identity of each respondent but their identity is confidential to you, then all questionnaires will require a confidential unique identifier. Names and addresses should not appear on the questionnaire itself. If, however, your survey is anonymous, then you cannot know the identity of any of your respondents and none of your questionnaires should have an identifier.

Instructions

It is crucial to include instructions on the questionnaire, in terms of ticking boxes, circling numbers, allocating priority order to a list, etc. If you are doing a postal survey or a questionnaire for self-completion, you will need clear instructions for the respondent. Alternatively, if using interviewers, you will need to provide them with instructions in terms of filtering and what to read out, etc.

Unless you use a ready-made questionnaire such as the SF36 or the GHQ, you will have to design your own. The style and content of a questionnaire will depend very much on your research question and your aims and objectives. A very structured interview or postal questionnaire will contain a greater proportion of closed questions with pre-coded answers, whereas a questionnaire or topic guide for use in a semi-structured interview will contain more open-ended questions.

Closed questions

A closed question is one where the possible answers are defined in advance and so the respondent is limited to one of the pre-coded responses given. For example, if you were to ask an asthma patient:

'Which of the following types of inhaler do you currently use?'
(INTERVIEWER TO READ OUT)

A dry powder inhaler	1
A metered-dose inhaler or	2
A breath-activated metered-dose inhaler	3

This is an example of a closed question, where the possible pre-codes would be read out or shown to the respondent on a card. The choice of answers is limited to those shown on the card.

Open-ended questions

An open-ended question does not constrain possible responses. For example, you could ask the same patient:

'How does having asthma affect your daily life?'

In this open-ended question, the respondent is allowed to interpret the question in their own way. They could, for instance, choose to talk about how having asthma interferes with their work, or how they can't go jogging in the winter or how they feel using an inhaler in front of schoolfriends. The answers you get back will be very rich in details, but it may be difficult to compare the responses over a large number of subjects because the question is not very directed. We haven't specified to the respondents, in this case, which areas of their lives we are interested in.

A problem with asking an open-ended question of lots of people is that it can produce lots of different answers, which can be difficult and time-consuming to code.

Partial pre-coding

This can be partially solved by using an open-ended question with partial pre-coding. There may be questions that we wish to ask in an open-ended manner so that we are not leading the respondents in any way, but nevertheless we can anticipate some of the possible responses. Potential responses can be anticipated by:

- carrying out a pilot study
- assessing previous studies
- guessing.

The important point to note is that the pre-codes listed do not need to be exhaustive; we can always allow for an 'other, please specify' option to catch the response which we hadn't thought of in advance. An example of an open-ended question with partial pre-coding would be:

'What do you think is the cause of your asthma?'
(INTERVIEWER INSTRUCTIONS) DO NOT READ OUT, CIRCLE ALL THAT APPLY

Air pollution	1
Traffic pollution/cars/exhaust fumes	2
Pollen	3
Dust/dust mites	4
Pets/dog/cat	5
Stress	6
Work/occupation	7
Certain foods/dairy products	8
Inherited from parents	9
Other, please specify _____	

In this case we have anticipated some of the most likely answers, but we have also allowed for the respondents to give answers which we hadn't thought of in advance. So, although some content analysis is still required, the overall amount is still reduced. This will save time in the analysis. This type of open-ended question can be asked in an interview situation, either face-to-face or over the telephone. With self-completion

> **Box 4.2 Definition**
>
> **Content analysis** is the systematic analysis of text or conversational transcripts to identify and group common themes.

questionnaires, the respondents would be able to see the pre-codes which could influence their choice of answer.

Coding

As you can see from the above, wherever possible we need to allocate a numeric code to each possible answer. This is so that the answers can be entered into a computer for data analysis. It is generally easier to specify the codes in advance where you can anticipate the possible answers, as in closed questions. Obviously with open-ended questions it may not be possible to anticipate all the possible answers. You will therefore have to code the open-ended questions as your questionnaires are returned. Some questions ask for numerical data, for instance: 'How old are you?' or 'How many times have you visited your GP in the last month?'. With questions like this you do not need to pre-code the answer; simply leave a blank box into which to enter the exact number.

The coding of other questions which include ordered categories, particularly those using bands or scales, is straightforward. For instance, if you ask the question:

'How long ago is it since you last saw a dentist?'
    Within the last month   1
    More than a month ago but within the last six months   2
    More than six months ago but within the last year   3
    More than a year ago   4

You can see we have allocated each possible answer a numeric code. The important thing to note, however, is that the answers are in a particular order, thus the codes given to each answer reflect this order. The gaps between each code, however, are not equal. This is known as *ordinal* data.

Finally we come to *nominal* data. Nominal data is where the codes allocated to the categories are purely nominal, i.e. the numbers themselves do not mean anything numerically, neither is there any sort of order implied by the numbers. The codes are there purely to act as numeric labels for each of the discrete categories.

So, for example, we might ask on a questionnaire:

'Are you male or female?'
    Male   '1' or 'M'
    Female   '2' or 'F'

The codes '1' and '2' do not mean anything numerically, they just signify that there are two different groups.

> **Box 4.3 Definition**
>
> **Ordinal data** is composed of categories which can be placed in an order. However, the gaps between each value are not necessarily of equal size.

> **Box 4.4 Definition**
>
> **Nominal data**, also known as categorical data, is a set of unordered categories. Codes are assigned on an arbitrary basis and have no numeric meaning.

Exercise 6

State whether the following questions are open-ended or closed:

1. 'How old are you?'
2. 'What is your name?'
3. 'What is your occupation?'
4. 'Would you say that traffic pollution has a direct effect on the number of people getting asthma attacks?'
   (READ OUT)
   'Yes, or No?'
5. 'At home do you have a pillow with a synthetic or a feather filling or both?'
6. 'Do you use a duvet at night?'
   (READ OUT)
   'Yes, or No?'
7. 'Does this have a synthetic or a feather filling?'
8. 'Do you own a furry pet?'
9. 'Do you own a dog or a cat?'
10. 'How many times a day do you use an inhaler?'
    (READ OUT)
    'Never'
    'Once a day'
    'Twice a day'
    'Three times a day'
    'Four or more times a day'

Question wording

The wording of your questions is all-important, as it has a direct impact on the outcome. Keep your questions simple, and use words that are easily understood by lay people. Avoid jargon, especially medical jargon. For instance, patients will not know that 'MI' means a heart attack and they may misinterpret the word 'drug', so use 'prescribed medicine' instead. Carry out the readability tests such as the Fog Index (see Appendix 1) and the Flesch Reading Ease Score (see page 103).

It is important to ensure that questions are not too long and that they don't contain several questions in one sentence, which will only confuse the respondent. For example,

'Does having asthma restrict the type of work and sporting activities that you can do?'

If the answer were 'Yes', what would it mean?

Avoid using ambiguous words and questions. Try not to assume anything about the respondent and avoid asking leading questions.

'We know that cigarette smoking can make asthma worse. How many cigarettes do you smoke a day?' or
'Do you think the fumes from car exhausts are the main cause of asthma?'

Producing comparable data

You may want to compare your findings with previous studies. If so, it is important that you use directly comparable wording. Questionnaire design is one area where it does not always pay to be creative. Many routine questions that you wish to ask will have been refined, tested and validated by other organisations already. For example, if you want to ask a question on ethnic origin, consider using the question used in the census by the OPCS, which has been thoroughly tested.

When collecting numeric data, try wherever possible to collect the data at the most detailed level you will need. For example, if you wish to record age, then do not present the respondents with age bands, rather ask them to give their exact ages. This will provide you with data at an interval level, rather than an ordinal level, which means that you can describe the data more fully. In this instance you would be able to describe the mean average age as well as the median, rather than the median alone. Interval level data also enable you to use more discriminating statistical tests.

Box 4.5   Definition

Interval data are measured on a scale where the distance between each point is equal.

On the other hand, if you want to ask about data that may be sensitive, such as income, or, if you think that the respondent will be unable to be accurate about the data,

> **Box 4.6 Definition**
>
> The **mean** is a measure of central tendency. It is calculated by summing all the values and dividing this by the number of cases to produce a mean average.

> **Box 4.7 Definition**
>
> The **median** is a measure of central tendency. If all the values are placed in order, the median is the midpoint or middle value.

then it is preferable to ask the question with potential answers in banded groups. This will generate data at an ordinal level, which may be less useful, but avoids spurious accuracy.

For instance, when asking questions about frequency of activity such as: 'When did you last visit your GP to discuss your asthma?' or 'How often do you use your "blue" inhaler on an average day?', it is important you use pre-codes wherever possible, because otherwise some of the answers may be so vague or wide-ranging that you will be unable to collate or compare the responses.

The question: 'When did you last visit your GP to discuss your asthma?' could be pre-coded as follows:

In the last week	1
In the last 2–4 weeks	2
More than a month ago	3
More than six months ago	4
More than a year ago	5
Can't remember	6

Exercise 7

Which of the following questions could be used in a survey of obesity? If a question could not be used, state why it is unsuitable.

1. Do you weigh more or less than ten stone?
2. Do you consider yourself to be obese?
3. Are you fat?
4. Do you consider yourself to be overweight?
5. Do you have a regular, balanced diet?
6. Do you ever take drugs to control your weight?
7. Has your GP ever prescribed medicine to control your weight?
8. What was the name of the drug prescribed, its dosage and how many times a day?
9. How many times a year do you start a diet?
10. What is your weight and height?

Question order

As a rule, it is best to move from the general to the particular when designing a questionnaire. Try to start with general fact-finding questions which are easily understood and will apply to everyone. These can act as a warm-up. Then move onto more specific questions, which may filter people into different questions. Certain personal questions, such as age, social class and ethnicity, may be left until later, near the end of the questionnaire, when a level of rapport has been established. Likewise, embarrassing or sensitive questions may be best left until nearer the end. As with in-depth interviews, the questionnaire should 'flow'.

The order of the questions is a particularly important issue to consider when planning a self-completion or postal survey. Although respondents may choose to look ahead, you must consider what the cumulative impact of each question is on the next.

Because you cannot assume anything about the respondent, it is inevitable that the questionnaire will need to contain certain filters and instructions to either the respondent or the interviewer as to where to go next. For instance:

Q3 Do you smoke cigarettes?
    Yes   1   If **Yes**, go to Q4
    No   2   If **No**, go to Q5
Q4 How many cigarettes do you smoke a day?
    1   1
    2–5   2
    6–10   3
    11–20   4
    21–30   5
    31–40   6
    41 or more   7

Overall try to keep the question topics in a logical order. It may be best to reflect the chronological order of events if necessary, but avoid over-complicated filtering, especially in self-completion questionnaires, because some respondents will be unable to follow it.

Exercise 8

In which order would you place the following questions in a self-administered questionnaire in a survey of stress amongst GPs?

1   Is stress affecting your personal life?
2   In which practice do you work?
3   Which is the best way of coping with stress?
4   How many surgeries a week do you have?

Dealing with sensitive questions

Apart from leaving sensitive questions to near the end of the questionnaire, there are other ways of trying to elicit an honest answer.

It is possible to introduce a question by reference to the activity of others, such as: 'Not everybody uses their inhalers as often as their doctors have told them to for a variety of reasons. Do you use your inhaler as often as your doctor has told you to?'

It may also be possible to use indirect questioning by referring to a third person before asking the respondent directly.

Using scales in questionnaires

One way of ensuring that a question is asked in a fair and balanced way is by the use of scales. Scales will also assist in measuring the strength of attitude/feeling rather than simply 'Yes' or 'No', 'Agree' or 'Disagree'.

It should be remembered, however, that a scale is not a precise measure of an attitude, merely a way of assessing relative measures. There are a variety of different scales to choose from.

Likert scale

The Likert scale is one of the most commonly used scales. Respondents are presented with one or more attitudinal statements and asked to score each statement on a multi-point scale. For instance,

'To what extent do you agree with the following statements?'

Statements	Strongly agree 5	Agree 4	Neither agree or disagree 3	Disagree 2	Strongly disagree 1
Traffic pollution is a major cause of asthma					
People with asthma who smoke a lot are more likely to have worse asthma					
I believe that the medicine prescribed for me by my doctor works well					

This is an example of a five-fold Likert scale; it is also possible to have a seven-fold Likert scale. Likert scales are very popular with researchers, and sometimes they succumb to a temptation to sum the results of all the scales into a single score. This can be potentially misleading.

There is some evidence to indicate that respondents may be more likely to disagree with a negative statement than agree with a positive statement (Cohen *et al.* (1996) *BMJ.* **313**: 841–44). So you need to think very carefully about how you word your statements and ensure that they are comparable with any other key studies with which you may want to compare your findings.

Semantic differential scale

Developed by Osgood in 1957, *semantic differential scales* are used to rate individual statements, on a number of different dimensions. For example:

'Do you think that the medicine that the doctor has prescribed for your asthma:

works well	1	2	3	4	5	doesn't work
is safe						is dangerous
has no side effects						has strong side effects
is pleasant to take						is unpleasant
is convenient						is inconvenient

Semantic differential scales only work well when the concepts at either end of the scale are mutually exclusive. If the respondent feels that they could select both ends of the scale, then the scale is impossible to answer. It is therefore very important to pilot the scales carefully.

Visual analogue scales

As an alternative to a verbal scale, a *visual analogue scale* is simply a way of asking respondents to indicate their choice visually or spatially. For instance:

'Do you think that traffic pollution has a bad effect on your asthma?'
Please place a cross on the line below.

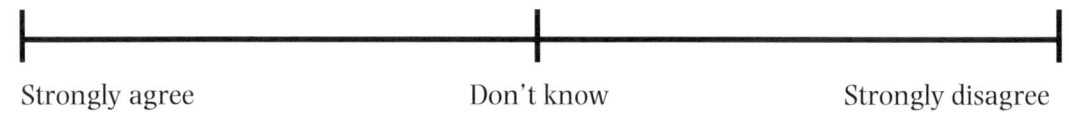

|─────────────────────────┼─────────────────────────|
Strongly agree   Don't know   Strongly disagree

A visual analogue scale is very difficult to interpret and is not recommended.

Ranking

A further way of getting respondents to express attitudes is by using ranking.

Respondents could be given a list of items on a show card and asked to rank them verbally, or they could be given a number of cards, each with an item on, and be asked to sort the cards into rank order, such as:

'Which of these items do you think has the worst effect on your asthma?',

followed by

'and the next'

and so on until all the items have been placed in rank order. For example:

Exercise
Traffic pollution
Stress
Diet
Pollen

Alternatively the respondents could be asked to allocate the numbers 1–5 beside each category.

Indices

Sometimes discrete questions are combined to create some kind of aggregate or composite score or index. Indices are tricky things to create because it is difficult to know what level of weighting should be assigned to each discrete element of the questionnaire. Researchers often make the mistake of treating the final score as interval data rather than ordinal data.

Pilot study

Before you can embark on the main stage of fieldwork, it is crucial that the draft questionnaire is piloted. You should never use a questionnaire which has not been piloted, particularly if the questionnaire is designed for self-completion and there will be nobody around to clear up misunderstandings. A pilot stage will enable you to ensure that:

- all the relevant issues are included
- the order is correct
- ambiguous or leading questions are identified
- your pre-codes are correct

- you have not forgotten or omitted some issue which is really important to the respondent.

The ideal situation is to test the questionnaire on a small number of respondents who are the same type as those in your sampling frame; between 5–50 respondents, depending upon the final sample size. However, if the real subjects are difficult to access or few in number, then you may have to test the questionnaire on slightly different subjects. At the very minimum you could try out the questionnaire on your colleagues or friends. This will at least allow you to see if the filtering and order is correct. Do remember, however, that if the questionnaire is destined for members of the public that you should test the questionnaire out on a lay person in preference to a professional colleague. Jargon which you use on a day-to-day basis may completely baffle members of the general public!

Using questionnaires in postal surveys

Postal surveys are a useful option to consider when selecting your method. They are usually cheaper and quicker than personal interviewing, especially if the sample is large. For any postal survey, regardless of the sample size, you must allow at least six weeks for the first wave of questionnaires to be returned, and another four weeks for each successive mailing. As with telephone interviewing, a postal survey is useful if your respondents are widely distributed. However, due to the lack of personal contact between the respondent and the researcher, the design and layout of the questionnaire is all-important. Given the popularity of postal surveys in primary care, we have included here a very practical section on how to conduct a postal survey.

Practical aspects of carrying out postal surveys

The questionnaire must be totally self-contained and self-explanatory. This means questionnaires with very complex flows and routing are not suitable. Any instructions on routing through the questionnaire, for example,

'if the answer to Q2 is YES, go to Q6',

need to be clearly stated. Sometimes the use of coloured arrows may help this process.

A questionnaire for self-completion must look inviting and user-friendly. If it appears too complex or too long, respondents simply will not bother. Obviously you need to be sure that your sampling frame has a sufficient literacy level before you can consider the use of a postal survey. If you think that your target population is likely to have a low literacy level, choose another method. (Note: the average questionnaire circulated by academics in the UK requires a reading age of 19.)

However, even with a literate population, it is necessary to cater for the lowest common denominator. Never use lengthy, complicated words when simple words will do.

Be careful to avoid professional jargon and try to use a lay person's language wherever possible when addressing the general public. Test the literacy level of the questionnaire first using the Fog Index or the Flesch Reading Ease Score.

> **Box 4.8 Definition**
>
> The **Fog Index** is a calculation used to assess the required reading age of written material (see Appendix 1 for details).

> **Box 4.9 Definition**
>
> The **Flesch Reading Ease** computes readability based on the average number of syllables per word and the average number of words per sentence. Scores range from 0 (zero) to 100. Standard writing usually scores between 60 and 70. The higher the score, the greater the number of people who can easily understand the document. (The Flesch Reading Ease Score, along with other readability statistics, is automatically calculated when using Microsoft Word software.)

If you are doing a survey of elderly people, then you may wish to consider increasing the size of the typeface used in the questionnaire.

The length of the questionnaire has to be carefully considered when conducting a postal survey, but if the subject matter is of sufficient interest to the respondent, then length is less important.

It is possible to achieve high response rates with a postal questionnaire provided you adhere to the following points:

- the subject matter must be of interest to the respondent and not too sensitive
- the sampling frame must be up to date
- you must carry out two waves of mailings
- you must provide a pre-paid self-addressed envelope for the replies
- you must reassure the respondents of their confidentiality in a covering letter
- the questionnaire must be well laid out, not too complicated and self-explanatory
- you must allow sufficient time for the responses – ideally four to six weeks
- you do not mail over holiday periods, such as Christmas.

All mailed questionnaires should be accompanied by a covering letter. This letter will need to include:

- who you are and your role in the survey
- what the survey is about and its potential benefits
- why the respondent has been selected
- reassurance for the respondent of their confidentiality or anonymity (for example, you could say: 'All the answers will be grouped together so that it will not be possible to identify your individual answers from the findings')

- details of where to return the questionnaire and a number to ring if they want to check the status of the survey.

> **Box 4.10 Definition**
>
> An **anonymous survey** is one in which respondents are not allocated ID numbers and cannot be identified in any way. Sometimes very sensitive topics require anonymous rather than confidential surveys.

> **Box 4.11 Definition**
>
> A **confidential survey** is one in which the respondents cannot be identified except with a unique ID number used to link responses back to an individual.

Other points to consider to increase response rates include:

- use of coloured paper
- sponsorship, for example a covering letter signed by somebody influential, such as a local GP
- using stamps rather than a franked envelope
- advance warning, using a letter or postcard
- using a personally addressed covering letter
- using small incentives such as vouchers, stamps, pens, donations to charity. (You need to be aware that a Local Ethics Research Committee may view an incentive as an unfair inducement to participate, so your incentive should not be too generous.)

Postal survey reminders

If two waves of mailing are proposed, it is necessary to make an estimate of the likely response rate to the first wave when deciding on the total number of questionnaires and envelopes required. Use Table 4.2 to guide your decision and remember that:

- every questionnaire will require two envelopes; one to be sent out and one for the reply
- everybody who has not replied to the first mailing will need to be sent a reminder letter, plus a questionnaire, plus a reply envelope.

For instance, if we mail 100 respondents and get responses initially from 40%, we will need to mail reminders to 60 people. So, in total we would require 160 questionnaires to achieve a response rate of 50%.

Table 4.2

Response rate	No. of questionnaires per 100 sample members	No. of envelopes per 100 sample members
50%	160	320
60%	150	300
70%	140	280
80%	130	260
90%	120	240

However, if our initial response rate is higher, e.g. 80%, we would only need to send reminders to 20 people to achieve a response rate of 90%. If we can estimate the response rate in advance, we can minimise the number of questionnaires and envelopes required. A pilot study or an assessment of previous studies may help you to decide on your anticipated response rate.

Data analysis

Finally we need to consider the analysis of the data. It is all too easy to busy oneself with the questionnaire design and data collection and not give any thought to the analysis stage. However, it is actually crucial to think about the analysis very early on. It is important to establish the exact data type of the main outcome measures, e.g. nominal, ordinal, or interval. The data type in turn determines which type of statistical test is most appropriate, and this in turn has implications for the required sample size.

Once the data have been assigned a numerical code, as discussed earlier, they need to be entered into the computer software that you will be using for data analysis. This is likely to be SPSS or Epi Info (see the Trent Focus research volume *Statistical Analysis in Primary Care*, Chapters 3 and 4 'An introduction to using SPSS' and 'An introduction to using Epi Info'). Once the data have been entered, it is necessary to check the data for errors and typos. Although it is possible to carry out some simple hand counts and therefore avoid computers, this approach is really not recommended. If your survey consists of more than 20 cases and you want to cross-tabulate the answers to two or more questions, it becomes practically impossible to do this by hand.

Once you are satisfied that the data you have entered onto the computer are correct, you will probably want to start your analysis by requesting basic frequencies. These are simple counts of the number of individuals answering each question. The next stage is to request *cross-tabulations* or *contingency tables*, which enable you to analyse the way that answers to one question might vary from answers to another question. For example:

We can see in Table 4.3 that there would be a difference in the consulting behaviour between men and women. However, just by looking at this we cannot tell if this difference is statistically significant. The next stage is to apply some statistical test to the data to see

Table 4.3 Gender by consultation with GP in last year

	Male	Female	Total no.
Consulted GP in last year	52	87	139
Not consulted GP in last year	57	13	70
Total no.	109	100	209

if there is a statistically significant difference between men and women in our sample in terms of consultations. In this particular example, the appropriate test to use would be a Chi-Square Test because both variables are nominal. It is important to understand that the most appropriate statistical test is likely to depend upon the type of data you are collecting and the number of groups that you are comparing. It is not possible to cover the statistical tests in detail here and you are advised to consult the Trent Focus research volume *Statistical Analysis in Primary Care* for further details.

The important point to remember is that you do not need to know how to calculate these tests by hand because the computer will do this for you. However, you do need to know which is the appropriate test to request and how to interpret the answer.

Exercise 9

Now consider your own research question and aims and objectives.

1. If a survey is a possible option, think about what type of methodology you might use and why.
2. Now think about some of the key questions that you might want to ask, and write these down.
3. A pilot study is essential in planning a survey. Write down how you would carry out a pilot study and why.
4. How would you go about selecting your subjects for interview in a pilot study and why?
5. What steps might you take to increase your response rate in the main stage of your fieldwork?

Summary

In this chapter we have concentrated on five main areas: why surveys are useful; different methods of how to carry out a survey; how to use questionnaires; aspects of questionnaire design; and using questionnaires in a postal survey.

You should by now be able to describe the advantages and disadvantages of the following methods:

- face-to-face interviews
- telephone interviews

- postal surveys
- self-completion questionnaires, including ready-made instruments.

You should be able to list the factors which may increase participation and/or response rate. You should understand the difference between open-ended and closed questions and know what a pre-code is. You should also be able to distinguish between a structured and a semi-structured questionnaire. As you will recall, a structured questionnaire with a majority of closed questions with pre-coded answers is appropriate when trying to directly compare the responses of a large number of people, whereas a semi-structured questionnaire will allow you to ask more open-ended questions which are rich in detail but more difficult to analyse and compare.

Remember when designing your questionnaire to avoid:

- using ambiguous or multiple questions
- using double negatives
- using long, complicated sentences or jargon
- using leading questions.

Finally, you should be able to list the factors which may increase participation and/or response rate.

Answers to exercises

Exercise 1

1. The ability to carry out a longer interview on a more complex topic, with complicated filtering; a higher response rate; the ability to use visual aids and prompts; the opportunity to develop a rapport.
2. Labour intensive for large samples; time-consuming; difficult to contact people at home.

Exercise 2

1. Easier to contact geographically-spread respondents; may be easier to contact professionals; can be cheaper and quicker than a face-to-face survey.
2. Not appropriate if sampling frame do not all have equal access to a telephone; sampling frame – even those with a telephone may be ex-directory; cannot use visual aids; interview may be impersonal; interview length is limited.

Exercise 3

1. Not labour intensive, possible to mail a large sample, and therefore may be cheaper than face-to-face or telephone; gives people opportunity to answer question in their

own time (they may need to refer to documents, etc); useful for a widely distributed sample.
2. Possibly lower response depending on topic and motivation; usually takes much longer, need to give people sufficient time to reply and send out mailers; not suitable for people with literacy problems.

Exercise 4

1. Stratified random sample. The sample is stratified because the sample has been selected to ensure that two different groups are represented.
2. Disproportionate stratified random sample. This sample is stratified to ensure that patients from the two different groups are picked up, however the two groups are selected, so that they are equal in size and are not representative of the patient base.
3. Quota. The sample is not randomly selected, but the respondents are selected to meet certain criteria.
4. Convenience. The sample is not randomly selected and no quotas are applied.
5. Systematic sample.
6. Cluster sample. The patients are selected only from certain wards.

Exercise 5

1. The researchers used a convenience sampling approach, i.e. they selected people on the basis that they were easy to access. Respondents were therefore self-selected.
2. The sampling method used was non-random.
3. The advantage of this approach was that they were able to obtain the views of a large number of people very quickly and easily with little expense.
4. Unfortunately the convenience sample approach means that the sample is not representative of the population of individuals with asthma. Because a large part of the survey is made up of people attending in surgery and pharmacies, the sample will tend to over-represent those individuals requiring the most treatment. It will also over-represent those individuals who are most interested in expressing their opinions.
5. The sample achieved was very large because it was self-selected, and therefore the researchers would have had little control over how many people participated.

Exercise 6

1. Open-ended.
2. Open-ended.
3. Open-ended.
4. Closed.
5. Closed.
6. Closed.
7. Closed.
8. Closed, but will probably attract some strange answers and questions!
9. Closed.
10. Closed.

Exercise 7

1. Does not provide all possible alternatives. What happens if the respondent weighs exactly ten stone?
2. The term 'obese' is jargon and not all respondents would understand its true meaning. (One lady who was told that she was obese by her GP thought he told her that she was a 'beast'.) A preferable term would be overweight.
3. Firstly the term 'fat' is derogatory and should not be used at all. This is also two questions in one.
4. Acceptable.
5. Ambitious and vague. What is meant by regular? What is meant by balanced? The question is too subjective.
6. Open to misinterpretation. The term 'drug' has a different meaning in lay use compared to its clinical definition.
7. Acceptable.
8. Three questions in one.
9. A leading question and assumes that the respondent uses diets.
10. Two questions in one.

Exercise 8

The correct order is 2, 4, 1, 3.

Exercise 9

Since this exercise is based on a self-selected example it is not possible to provide specific answers to the questions. You should, however, draw on the guidelines in the text when approaching them.

Further reading

Carter Y and Thomas C (eds) (1997) *Research Methods in Primary Care*. Radcliffe Medical Press, Oxford.

Crombie I and Davies H (1996) *Research in Health Care*. John Wiley & Sons Ltd., Chichester.

Lygeard S (1991) The Questionnaire as a Research Tool. *Family Practice*. **8**: 84–91.

Moser C and Kalton G (1990) *Survey Methods in Social Investigation*. Gower, Hants.

Oppenheim A (1992) *Questionnaire Design, Interviewing and Attitude Measurement*. Pinter Publishers Ltd., London.

Robson C (1993) *Real World Research*. Blackwell, Oxford.

Sapsford R and Jupp V (1996) *Data Collection and Analysis*. Sage Publications, London.

Stone D (1993) How to design a questionnaire. *BMJ*. **307**:1264–66.

For further information on ready-made health indices

Bowling A (1995) *Measuring Disease*. Open University Press, Buckingham.

Bowling A (1995) *Measuring Health: A Review of Quality of Life Measurement Scales*. Open University Press, Buckingham.

Hutchinson A, McColl E, Christie M and Riccalton C (1996) *Health Outcome Measures in Primary and Out-Patient Care*. Harvard Academic Publishers, The Netherlands.

Wilkin D, Hallam L and Dogget M (1994) *Measures of Need and Outcome for Primary Health Care*. Oxford University Press, Oxford.

Appendix 1: The Fog Index

The Fog Index was developed by an American, Robert Gunning, as a way of quickly checking the readability of text. It is calculated in the following way:

1. Take a piece of text of about 100 words.
2. Divide the number of words by the number of sentences. This gives the average number of words per sentence.
3. Count up the number of words of three syllables or more in the passage, e.g. 'ibuprofen', 'infarction', 'leukaemia'. Don't count words that are: capitalised, combinations of short words, made into three syllables by the addition of -ed or -es, e.g. admitted. This gives you the percentage of 'hard' words in the passage.
4. Add the average number of words per sentence to the percentage of 'hard' words in the passage. Multiply by 0.4 to get the Fog Index.

The Fog Index aims to show the number of years of education which the reader needs to have had to understand the text. So text with an index of 12 should be clear to a reader who left school at 17 (assuming he started at age 5). Remember that the Fog Index is just a guide.

CHAPTER FIVE

Using interviews in a research project

Nigel Mathers, Nick Fox and Amanda Hunn

Introduction

The interview is an important data-gathering technique involving verbal communication between the researcher and the subject. Interviews are commonly used in survey designs and in exploratory and descriptive studies. There are a range of approaches to interviewing, from completely unstructured, in which the subject is allowed to talk freely about whatever they wish, to highly structured, in which the subject responses are limited to answering direct questions.

The quality of the data collected in an interview will depend on both the interview design and on the skill of the interviewer. For example, a poorly-designed interview may include leading questions or questions that are not understood by the subject. A poor interviewer may consciously or unconsciously influence the responses that the subject makes. In either circumstance, the research findings will be influenced detrimentally.

It is often assumed that if someone is clinically trained and used to dealing with patients that this is sufficient training to carry out interviews with patients and others for research purposes. Although there are some areas of overlap in terms of the basic communication skills required, it should be acknowledged that for research some different skills are required. The context is also important, since in a clinical setting there is a particular relationship between a patient and clinician. It is possible that in this routine setting the patient would not be prepared to answer all the questions in a completely honest manner. So it may well be worthwhile thinking about the interview from the respondent's point of view and considering carefully who would be the most appropriate person to conduct the interview and in what setting. There may be a conflict of roles, for example therapeutic versus research, or even an unconscious adoption of roles that could affect the quality of the data collected.

Having successfully completed the work in this chapter, you will be able to:

- describe the skills required to undertake a structured, semi-structured or unstructured interview
- summarise the advantages and disadvantages of face-to-face and telephone interviews
- outline the ways in which different types of interview data can be analysed.

Types of interview

The interview design and question phrasing will influence the depth and freedom with which a subject can respond. Some interviews encourage lengthy and detailed replies, while others are designed to elicit short and specific responses. The degree of structure imposed on an interview will actually vary along a continuum, but it is useful to think of three main types: structured, semi-structured and unstructured.

Structured or standardised interviews

Structured interviews enable the interviewer to ask each respondent the same questions in the same way. A tightly structured schedule of questions is used, very much like a questionnaire. The questions contained in the questionnaire will have been planned in advance, sometimes with the help of a pilot study to refine the questions.

The questions in a structured interview may be phrased in such a way that a limited range of responses is elicited. For example: 'Do you think that health services in this area are excellent, good, average or poor?'

This is an example of a closed question where the possible answers are defined in advance so that the respondent is limited to one of the pre-coded responses.

It is not unusual for otherwise structured interviews to contain a few open-ended questions. 'Catch-all' final questions are common, for example: 'Do you have anything more to add?' These questions are useful in helping to capture as much information as possible, but they increase the amount of time required for analysing the interview findings.

Semi-structured interviews

Semi-structured interviews involve a series of open-ended questions based on the topic areas the researcher wants to cover. The open-ended nature of the question defines the topic under investigation, but provides opportunities for both interviewer and interviewee to discuss some topics in more detail. If the interviewee has difficulty answering a question or provides only a brief response, the interviewer can use cues or prompts to encourage the interviewee to consider the question further. In a semi-structured interview, the interviewer also has the freedom to probe the interviewee to elaborate on the original response or to follow a line of inquiry introduced by the interviewee. An example would be:

Interviewer: 'I'd like to hear your thoughts on whether changes in government policy have changed the work of the doctor in general practice. Has your work changed at all?'
Interviewee: 'Absolutely! The workload has increased for a start.'
Interviewer: 'In what way has it increased?'

Semi-structured interviews are useful when collecting attitudinal information on a large scale, or when the research is exploratory and it is not possible to draw up a list of possible pre-codes because little is known about the subject area. However, analysing the interview data from open questions is more problematic than when closed questions are used, as work must be done before (often diverse) responses from subjects can be compared.

Well-planned and well-conducted semi-structured interviews are the result of rigorous preparation. The development of the interview schedule, conducting the interview and analysing the interview data all require careful consideration and preparation.

Unstructured or in-depth interviews

Unstructured interviews (sometimes referred to as 'depth' or 'in-depth' interviews) are so called because they have very little structure at all. The interviewer approaches the interview with the aim of discussing a limited number of topics, sometimes as few as one or two, and frames successive questions according to the interviewee's previous response. Although only one or two topics are discussed, they are covered in great detail. The interview might begin with the interviewer saying: 'I'd like to hear your views on GP commissioning'. Subsequent questions would follow from the interviewee's responses. Unstructured interviews are exactly what they sound like – interviews where the interviewer wants to find out about a specific topic but has no structure or preconceived plan or expectation as to how the interview will proceed.

Generally, a researcher will try to understand the informant's worldview in an unstructured interview. The relationship between the interviewer and the informant is important. Some characteristics of depth interviewing are that the researcher has a general purpose and may use a *topic guide*, but the informant provides most of the structure of the interview. Generally the researcher follows up on 'cues' or leads provided by the informant.

Face-to-face interviews

Face-to-face or personal interviews are very labour intensive, but can be the best way of collecting high-quality data. Face-to-face interviews are preferable: when the subject matter is very sensitive; if the questions are very complex; or if the interview is likely to be lengthy. Interviewing skills are dealt with in more detail later in this chapter.

Compared to other methods of data collection, face-to-face interviewing offers a greater degree of flexibility. A skilled interviewer can explain the purpose of the interview and encourage potential respondents to co-operate; they can also clarify questions, correct misunderstandings, offer prompts, probe responses and follow up on new ideas in a way that is just not possible with other methods.

Telephone interviews

Telephone interviews can be a very effective and economical way of collecting data where the sample to be contacted are all accessible via the telephone. They are not an appropriate method of data collection for a deprived population where telephone ownership is likely to be low or where respondents may be ex-directory. However telephone interviewing can be ideally suited to busy professional respondents, such as general practitioners, when the telephone numbers can be easily identified and timed appointments set up. Telephone interviews are also particularly useful when the respondents to be interviewed are geographically widely distributed.

One of the main disadvantages of a telephone interview is that it is difficult to incorporate visual aids and prompts and the respondents cannot read cards or scales. The length of a telephone interview is also limited, although this will vary with subject area and motivation. Nevertheless, it is possible to make prior appointments for a telephone interview and send stimulus material for the respondent to look at in advance. A prior appointment and covering letter may enhance the response rate and length of interview.

It is important to note that any findings derived from a telephone survey of the general population should be interpreted to take account of the non-responders who may not have access to a telephone or may be ex-directory.

Focus groups

Sometimes it is preferable to collect information from groups of people rather than from a series of individuals. Focus groups can be useful to obtain certain types of information, or when circumstances would make it difficult to collect information using other methods of data collection. They have been widely used in the private sector over the past few decades, particularly in market research, and are being increasingly used in the public sector.

Group interviews can be used when:

- limited resources prevent more than a small number of interviews to be undertaken
- it is possible to identify a number of individuals who share a common factor and it is desirable to collect the views of several people within that population subgroup

- group interaction among participants has the potential for greater insights to be developed.

Characteristics of a focus group

1. The recommended size of a group is 6–10 people. A smaller number than this limits the potential on the amount of collective information. A larger number makes it difficult for everyone to participate and interact.
2. Several focus groups should be run in any one research project. It would be wrong to rely on the views of just one group as it may be subject to internal or external factors of which the investigator is unaware. This can lead to idiosyncratic results. Individual groups may not work well: the members may be reluctant to participate or not interact well with each other and therefore limited insight will be gained. Sufficient groups should be run to provide adequate breadth and depth of information, but a small number of groups may achieve this, as few as three or four. There is no upper limit on the number of focus group interviews that could be held, although this will be limited by resources.
3. The members of each focus group should have something in common, characteristics which are important to the topic of investigation. For example, they may all be members of the same profession or they may work in the same team. They may all be patients at a practice or have experienced a similar health problem or be receiving similar treatment. Participants might or might not know each other. There are advantages and disadvantages to both.
4. Following on from point 3, focus groups are usually specially convened groups. It may be necessary or even desirable to use pre-formed groups, but difficulties may occur. This is usually due to the pre-existing purpose of the group, which can lead to the group having a particular perspective or bias which limits their potential for providing information, e.g. pressure groups or groups with some political basis.
5. Qualitative information is collected which makes use of participants' feelings, perceptions and opinions. Just as in individual interviews, data collection and analysis is time-consuming.
6. Using qualitative approaches requires certain skills. The researchers require a range of skills: group skills in facilitating and moderating, listening, observing and analysing.

When focus groups could be used

1. When little is known about the research topic and initial clues and insights are needed, e.g. the researcher wants to know about the professional culture of professions with which he is not familiar.
2. When there is a communication or understanding gap between groups or categories of people and the collection of data would be enhanced by facilitating some discussion between these groups, e.g. the views of both parents and teachers on how to provide health promotion for young people. Part of the discussion might

include the expectations that each group has of each other in terms of the type of information they expect young people to be provided with.
3. When the research team wants to collect ideas about how to deal with problems identified in an earlier stage of the research project, e.g. after identifying a need for a mobile Well-Woman or Well-Man clinic in rural areas, what sort of services should it provide or where are the geographical areas in most need.
4. When the method satisfies the requirements of key stakeholders. They may be more convinced by information collected from a larger sample than would be possible from individual interviews, yet value the depth of understanding which could not be achieved from questionnaires.
5. When the researcher wants to include the views of a larger number of people than would be feasible through individual interviews.

It is not advisable to use focus groups in emotionally charged settings where this type of discussion can intensify the conflict. It may be imprudent if the researcher cannot ensure the confidentiality of sensitive information. Nor is it acceptable to use focus groups unless the researcher is clear about the purpose and benefits of this method over other methods which may produce information which is better or more economical.

Interviewer tasks and skills

To conduct a good interview, interviewers need to be trained. This training includes familiarising a researcher with the skills of, for example, reflective questioning, summarising and controlling an interview.

So what are the requirements for a good interview? Well clearly, all interviewers need to appear unbiased, be systematic and thorough and offer no personal views. He or she also needs to be well informed on the purpose of the research interview and to be well prepared and familiar with the questionnaire or topic guide. In addition, he or she needs to be a good listener and all interviews should be private.

In carrying out a structured interview, it is important that the interviewer adheres closely to the interview instructions, namely:

- following the correct order and filtering throughout the questionnaire
- keeping personal opinions to oneself
- reading out pre-codes and prompts where instructed
- probing when necessary
- not reading out pre-codes for questions requiring spontaneous answers
- writing down open-ended responses in full.

Using a structured interview is a way of trying to ensure consistency between interviews. However, it is still important that interviewers are trained to administer the questionnaires and are well briefed on the interview topic, ensuring familiarity with some of the terms and jargon that may be contained in the answers.

> **Box 5.1   Definition**
>
> **Filtering** enables the interviewer or respondent to know which question to go to next. For example:
>
> - If yes to Q1, go to Q3
> - If no to Q1, go to Q2.

> **Box 5.2   Definition**
>
> A **prompt** is a prepared answer read out to the respondent by the interviewer.

> **Box 5.3   Definition**
>
> A **probe** is a follow-up question that is used after the respondent has given their first answer. It is used to elicit a more detailed response. Sometimes probes are general and non-directed. In contrast some probes are very specific, for example clarifying time of day.

Essentially an interviewer has four key tasks:

- to locate the respondent
- to obtain agreement to the interview
- to ask the questions
- to record the answers.

Locating the respondent

The location of respondents is determined by the sampling procedure, which should be agreed at the start of the study. In a quantitative study using a random sampling procedure, the interviewer does not have the discretion to decide whom to interview and must stick to a pre-determined list. The location and timing of the interview should be convenient for the interviewee. The interviewee should be told in advance how long the interview should take.

Obtaining agreement for the study

It is important that the interviewer seeks the informed consent of the respondent to participating in the study. In most cases, this should be obtained in writing. The interviewer has an important role in explaining why the study is necessary and converting waivers without coercion. Whilst it is possible to recruit respondents on the doorstep, it is preferable to invite them to participate in advance either in writing or by telephone. A written invitation on letter-headed paper explaining the purpose of the study can enhance the credibility of the study and increase response rates. Nevertheless such an invitation should be careful to explain that participation is entirely voluntary.

The interviewer must reassure the respondent of their confidentiality or anonymity, and inform them that their identities will not be revealed in the aggregated findings.

It is important that the interviewer introduces themselves, explains why the study is being done, why the respondent has been selected and what will happen to the interview data. Respondents should be encouraged to ask questions. All this will help the interviewer to establish a rapport with the respondent.

Asking the questions

Interviewers carrying out structured or semi-structured interviews for a quantitative study should:

- stick closely to any written instructions about filtering questions, what to read out etc.
- refrain from giving personal opinions
- be systematic and consistent in the way they interact with each respondent.

Recording the answers

In structured or semi-structured interviews, interviewers must record all answers carefully, distinguishing between questions which only allow one answer and multiple-response questions. Any verbatim answers need to be written down as accurately as possible.

In unstructured interviews, an interviewer would normally tape-record the discussion rather than attempt to get it all down on paper. This frees the interviewer to really listen to what is being said and to respond accordingly.

Finally, when ending the interview remember to give the respondent a contact telephone number in writing for the interviewer or study organiser. This gives some credibility to the study, enabling the respondent to check the status of the study if in doubt, or there may be something that the respondent wants to add or ask about.

Sources of error and bias in interviewing

Because of the personal nature of interviewing, the scope for introducing error and bias is quite large and can affect all the following stages of the interviewing process:

- asking the questions
- interpreting the answers

- recording the answers
- coding the answers.

Sources of interviewing error will affect a study randomly, i.e. in all directions, whereas sources of interviewing bias affect the study results systematically, i.e. in the same direction. Sources of error include:

1. Deviation from the written instructions on the questionnaire, e.g. not following the correct order of questions, not following the correct filters on the question routing, not using show cards with pre-coded answers, reading out pre-coded answers which were not to be read out, and changing the wording of the questions.
2. Interrogation error, which occurs when questions are phrased differently from one respondent to the next, e.g. asking: 'What is your age?' could produce a different response than asking 'How old are you?' Use of the word 'old' can result in some respondents giving a younger age.
3. Interpretation error, which occurs when the interviewer has to make a subjective judgement as to how to code an answer. This is most likely to happen when the potential answers are pre-coded and the interviewer has to attempt to squeeze the respondent's answer into an existing box.
4. Recording error. It is generally recognised that the more an interviewer has to write down, the more likely s/he is to make a mistake in the recording of that data. There is a tendency to abbreviate answers, not necessarily correctly.

Every effort should be made to reduce any possible error and bias, and so strengthen both the validity and reliability of the study.

Exercise 1

Write down how you think it might be possible to minimise interviewer error.

Preparing and conducting the interview

The interview schedule

Devising an interview schedule – the content of the interview – involves decisions about the following:

- what questions to ask
- how to phrase the questions
- breadth and depth of topics to be included
- question sequence.

The interview schedule will obviously depend on the purpose and focus of the research. However, there are a few guidelines that should be followed.

1. The questions must be answerable. There is no point in asking questions that the interviewee will not be able to answer because of lack of experience or knowledge.
2. Leading questions should be avoided. Asking a patient: 'Don't you agree that your treatment on the unit has been excellent?' is not acceptable as it encourages a particular response. The question would better be phrased as, 'Tell me what you think about your treatment on the unit'.
3. Semi-structured and unstructured interviews may be concerned with eliciting peoples' experiences, opinions and beliefs. Some questions will be designed to find out what interviewees actually know about a topic, other questions will focus on beliefs or views. Interviewees' responses may be based on first-hand experience or on what they have picked up from a third party. It is important that the interviewer checks out with the interviewee what perspective they are using in the response.
4. Interviews are time-consuming for the interviewee as well as the interviewer and as a courtesy, the interview should be kept to the minimum time necessary to deal with the topic. The interviewer should make sure that the key issues have been addressed and resist the temptation to get sidetracked. Recommended times for an interview varies from 20 to 40 minutes. It can be difficult to establish a rapport in too short a time, but conversely taking too long is unfair to the interviewee and interviews that take an hour or more are not really acceptable.
5. Avoid using words or phrases that the interviewee will not understand. Avoid using medical jargon with non-healthcare professionals.
6. Some words have different meanings for different people. For example, a question about the availability of exercise facilities in a geographical area might lead some people to think in narrow terms of exercise gyms and fitness centres, while others might include outdoor playing fields or even the possibilities for walks in the nearby countryside.
7. Similarly, be aware that some words are highly subjective and value laden. For example, a question about how 'good' or 'satisfactory' the local health services are should be followed up to ascertain what the interviewee means by 'good' or 'satisfactory'.
8. Some interviewees will be able to provide data about the full range of issues covered by the interview schedule, while others will have in-depth insights into some of the issues and little or no information on others. Careful use of prompts and probing should enable the interviewer to judge when a topic is worth exploring further and when to move on to the next topic.
9. Interviewees bring a range of perspectives with them. For example, a district nurse will answer a question on availability or access to services based on her experience with patients, but she may also have experience as a patient herself.
10. The first question in an interview should be something that interviewees will be able to answer without difficulty. This will help them to relax and encourage them to open up. Factual questions can be a useful starting point. Personal information about the interviewee can be asked at the beginning, provided the questions don't deal with very private or potentially sensitive or embarrassing issues.

11. The interview then moves into a discussion about the topics of particular interest. Responses to the main questions are extended through the use of supplementary questions designed to prompt or probe the interviewee.
12. The interviewer signals that the interview is nearing the end by techniques such as summarising or recapping the main points of the discussion. The interviewee is invited to correct anything that the interviewer appears to have misunderstood or to add any additional points.

Conducting the interview

Preparing for the interview

The interviewer requires good communication skills. Although it has been suggested that a semi-structured interview has the appearance of a discussion or a conversation, this is due to the skills of the interviewer in facilitating a relaxed, non-threatening atmosphere where interviewees feel comfortable to express themselves. Interviewers may require training before undertaking the interviews. Training should include:

- how to ask questions: phrasing and paralinguistics (voice tone and pitch, stress on particular words or phrases) can influence potential responses
- listening skills: indicating interest to build up rapport; listening to the answers of previous questions and using this in framing the next question; knowing when to wait and when to prompt
- negative reinforcement: the ability to intervene tactfully when the interviewee is going off at a tangent or going on for too long about a particular point.

Avoiding interviewer bias

The interviewer should avoid bringing their personal perspectives into the discussion. This can occur in the phrasing of questions, the use of prompts, and the selection of which responses to probe further. The interviewer should always concentrate on what the interviewees are saying and clarifying what they mean. The more time spent on active listening and the less time the interviewer spends talking, the less directive the interview will be and the less likelihood there is of bias being introduced.

Arranging the interview

Prospective interviewees may be invited to participate either in writing or by telephone. The invitation should indicate the purpose of the interview and what this will involve. It should be clear that participation is voluntary. Ethical issues such as whether interviewees' identities will remain anonymous to all but the researcher(s) and the confidentiality of data should be addressed. Once prospective interviewees have confirmed their willingness to take part, the date, time and place of the interview is arranged.

The meeting place should be convenient for the interviewee. Effort should be made to avoid interruption wherever possible and this can be helped by informing the interviewee in advance of how long the interview should take and making sure the interview takes place at the most convenient time.

Establishing rapport

Before commencing the interview the interviewer should take time to explain again the reason for the interview, including the aim of the research project and what will happen to the interview data. He or she should check whether the interviewee has any questions. Questions should be asked in a relaxed informal manner so that the interview appears more like a discussion or conversation. The interviewer must be aware of the effect of body language in indicating interest, encouraging the interviewee to talk, and maintaining a non-threatening atmosphere.

Conducting the interview

The interview should 'flow'. Beginning gently with factual questions and moving towards more personal questions later on can facilitate this. A gentle probe is necessary when the answer to a question is neither clear nor complete.

Some helpful techniques in conducting an interview are:

- don't interrupt; let respondents finish their train of thought
- follow up leads, i.e. respond to answers given, as some answers will lead onto the next question. (If the respondent gives an answer that you hadn't anticipated or even considered, follow this up first and ask questions about it before you forget it.)
- ask about both sides of the issue
- use reflective comments which give the respondent permission to continue to discuss and consider a particular topic.

Avoid double questions or being too helpful. It is generally felt that personal opinions should be avoided and care should be taken not to be led too far from the point. Having said this, there is a debate about the degree of empathy required to build trust and rapport with the respondent. Many qualitative interviewers feel that a degree of empathy is required to achieve a certain level of rapport and trust with the respondent and this may involve expressing some opinions of their own. For instance, Ann Oakley found whilst interviewing mothers before and after childbirth that it was impossible to abide by normal interviewing guidelines, and in order to gain the trust of her respondents she had to engage in normal conversations with them, often offering advice and information when asked (Oakley 1981). She felt that to do otherwise would have inhibited the degree of rapport between them. Some qualitative researchers take this to the extreme by immersing themselves in the culture prior to the interviewing stage. This is known as 'living the culture'.

Whilst the degree of empathy which can be shown in an unstructured interview is a debatable point, it is never appropriate to show disagreement or disapproval.

Body language

It is also important to try to pick up on non-verbal cues. Look at the respondent's posture: are they relaxed and comfortable or sitting perched on the edge of their seat? Look at the respondent's hands: what is she doing with them; is she biting her nails, holding her hand over her mouth whilst she speaks, or sitting on them? Is the interview emotionally distressing? The body language may indicate that there is more information to come.

Your own body language is important in making the respondent feel at ease by responding to their verbal and non-verbal cues. This is something we all usually do unconsciously.

Silences

Silences may be very telling. Do not feel uncomfortable with a silence in a qualitative interview. If you do, you may try to rush in and fill it quickly with another question. You need to give the respondent the opportunity and time to reflect and to add additional information. The length of the silence may be important and should be indicated in the final transcript.

Recording data

Interviewers have a choice of whether to take notes of responses during the interview or to tape-record the interview. The latter is preferable for a number of reasons. The interviewer can concentrate on listening and responding to the interviewee and is not distracted by trying to write down what has been said. The discussion flows because the interviewer does not have to write down the response to one question before moving on to the next. In note-taking there is an increased risk of interviewer bias because the interviewer is likely to make notes of the comments which make immediate sense or are perceived as being directly relevant or particularly interesting. Tape-recording ensures that the whole interview is captured and provides complete data for analysis so cues that were missed the first time can be recognised when listening to the recording. Lastly, interviewees may feel inhibited if the interviewer suddenly starts to scribble: they may wonder why what they have just said was of particular interest.

The ideal tape-recorder is small, unobtrusive and produces good-quality recording. An in-built microphone makes the participants less self-conscious. An auto-reverse facility is useful if the interview lasts longer than the recording time available on one side of the tape: this prevents an interruption in the flow of conversation. A tape-recorder with a counter facility can be useful when analysing the taped data.

Closing the interview

An in-depth interview can last between 40 minutes and three hours, depending on the level of interest generated in the topic. One of the most difficult things to do is to close an interview and one needs to develop a repertoire of signals to indicate it is the end. These can be as direct as switching off the tape-recorder (although clearly not in mid-sentence!), but there are more subtle techniques available (Mays and Pope 1995). Time should be taken to listen to the last remarks and any queries a subject may have should be dealt with then and there if possible.

Tips for in-depth interviewing
- be familiar with the aims and objectives of the research
- know your topic guide well; you may not get a chance to refer to it
- tape-record your interview if possible because you won't be able to write it all down
- reassure the respondent on the issue of confidentiality
- be a good listener and don't interrupt too much
- try to start with factual background questions and move gently towards more specific personal questions
- do not express your own personal opinions or appear biased – think in advance about your own prejudices, especially in the areas of sex, race, and age
- use probes when answers need further clarification, and respond to non-verbal cues
- transcribe the tape as soon as possible after the interview
- never underestimate the amount of time required for transcribing the tape and carrying out the analysis. A general rule of thumb is that for every hour of interview you have carried out, you will need to allow ten hours for the transcribing and analysis process.

The pilot study

In order to ensure that you have covered all the relevant issues, that your pre-codes are correct and that you have not forgotten or omitted some issue that is really important to the respondent, you will need to conduct a pilot study using your draft questionnaire.

The ideal situation is to test the questionnaire on a small number of respondents who are the same type as those in your sampling frame. Ideally you should test out your interview on between 10 and 50 respondents for a quantitative study. However, if the real subjects are difficult to access or few in number, then you may have to test the questionnaire on slightly different subjects. At the very minimum you could try out the questionnaire on your colleagues or friends. This will at least allow you to see if the filtering and order is correct.

It is essential that the interview be phrased in plain and clear language. If the subjects of your study are to be members of the public, you should pilot the interview with a lay person in preference to a professional colleague. You may be so familiar with medical terminology and jargon that you forget other people may not understand it.

Using interviews in a research project **127**

Exercise 2

Read the transcript below of a research interview between a practice nurse and a patient. Identify (by line number) those parts of the interview where the interviewer asked:

- leading questions
- ambiguous questions
- two questions in one sentence.

1. State how this may have influenced the outcome of the study.
2. Suggest ways in which the questions could have been better phrased.

The following is an extract from a qualitative interview between a practice nurse and a patient. The study aims to explore how parents decide to use primary care services when their children are ill.

```
 1  I   Interviewer: Thank you for agreeing to spare me some time for this interview.
 2      I'm doing a study of parents with small children – I'm interested in how they use
        their local general
 3      practitioner services.
 4  I   I'd like to ask you some questions about the times when your child has been ill.
 5      How old is she?
 6  R   Respondent: Six. She was six in June.
 7  I   Can you tell me about the last time she was ill?
 8  R   What do you mean by ill? How ill?
 9  I   Well, anything really, not necessarily ill enough to go to a doctor. I mean, eh, has
10      she had any colds or high temperatures or anything like that or more serious
        illness?
11  R   Yes.
12  I   She had 'em?
13  R   She had a bad cough and cold about two months ago.
14  I   And how did you handle that? Did you take her to the doctor?
15  R   Well, I didn't take her to the doctor straight away. I gave lots of Calpol and I
16      waited, and I tried to keep her cool, but then she seemed to get hotter and hotter
17      and eventually by night-time I decided that I had to call the doctor out.
18  I   What time was this?
19  R   About 3 am. She'd been awake all night and she'd been getting hotter and hotter
20      and I got more worried. You know how it is when you're worried.
21  I   You were worried about meningitis?
22  R   Yes, she was very poorly, so I called the doctor out.
23  I   So you asked for a home visit. How quickly did he come?
24  R   It was a woman, a different doctor. She came very quickly actually. I was surprised
25      she came so quickly. I thought that we would be waiting all night, you know. But
26      she was there within half an hour.
27  I   What did she do?
```

28 R Well she took Anna's temperature and, you know, she said she was OK. Not to
29   worry and that if we were still worried we should go to the GP in the morning.
30   I wanted some antibiotics but I didn't get any.
31 I So the next day did you take her to the GP or did you treat her yourself?
32 R Eh, yes.
33 I Sorry, did you treat her yourself?
34 R Well, I gave her some Calpol, but then I took her down to the health centre and
35   we saw Dr X and he examined her and I felt more reassured.
36 I Good. Was that reassurance important?
37 R Yes. I needed somebody to look at her properly and to listen to me.
38 I What about the time she was ill before that?
39 R (silence – respondent thinking) Well, I think she was ill around Christmas. She
40   had chickenpox.
41 I She must have felt pretty ill with that?
42 R No, actually. It hardly seemed to bother her. She was covered in spots, but she
43   carried on playing with her presents and she didn't like it when I told her she
      couldn't go to school.
44 I Did you take her to the doctor's?
45 R Yes, of course. As soon as I saw the spots. I took her straight down. And we saw
46   Dr X. He knew what it was straight away.
47 I So at what point did you decide to go to the doctor's?
48 R I'm not sure. I just wanted to know what the spots were. I wasn't worried cos
49   there was a lot of it about at the time.
50 I How did you decide whether to go to the doctor's or call out a doctor for a home
      visit?
51 R Well, it depends on the time of day and how worried you are.

Handling interview data

The way you analyse your interview data will depend on whether the data you have collected are predominantly quantitative (number-based) or qualitative (text-based). Let's look first at quantitative data analysis.

Analysis of quantitative data

Assuming that you had asked a number of questions of a large group of people, for instance over 20 respondents, then you are likely to want to use computer software to carry out your analysis. Most people use either SPSS or Epi Info to carry out their statistical analysis. SPSS is very user-friendly, but it can be very expensive to purchase. Epi Info, on the other hand, is freely available (for further details see the Trent Focus research volume *Statistical Analysis in Primary Care* Chapters 3 and 4, 'An introduction to using SPSS' and 'An introduction to using Epi Info').

Once you have gained access to either of these statistical packages you will need to define your variables and value labels, and then input the data. Once you have entered the data it is necessary to check for errors as it is very easy to type in the wrong figures. It is useful at this stage to print out some *frequencies*. These are simple counts of each of your main variables. So, for example, if one of your variables is the gender of the respondents, coded 1 and 2, then the frequencies command will calculate for you how many men and how many women were in your sample and reveal only entries outside the expected range.

The next stage is usually to carry out some simple cross-tabulations or contingency tables to compare responses to one question with another. So, for example, frequencies will enable you to see how many men and women you have in your sample and also how many smoke, but until you carry out a cross-tabulation you won't know how smoking varies by gender. For further details on quantitative data analysis see the Trent Focus research volume *Statistical Analysis in Primary Care*.

Analysis of qualitative data

If you have carried out a semi-structured or an in-depth interview, you will want to analyse the data using qualitative methods. It would be quite wrong to try and quantify the results of an in-depth interview. For instance, if you carried out ten in-depth interviews, you should not say that six out of the ten people interviewed took a particular viewpoint. Instead you should be looking at how and why the respondents differ in their views.

The first stage of qualitative analysis is to examine the transcripts of all your interviews. It is important that you get all the tapes of your interviews transcribed. It is much more difficult, if not impossible to try and do your analysis from the tapes alone. Using transcripts means that you pick up on the detail, including all those points that you might have forgotten. But don't forget to allow sufficient time to get the tapes transcribed. This can be a very painstaking process and you should never underestimate the amount of time that it can take.

Once you have all your transcripts together, you will need to carry out content analysis. This is really a systematic way of identifying all the main concepts which arise in the interviews, and then trying to categorise and develop these into common themes. It can be very confusing when you are faced with 14 long transcripts, but there are a number of practical ways of actually carrying out this process in a systematic way. To begin with you need to read through each transcript and make a note in the margin of main concepts or points of interest.

In order to identify the common themes and categories in the text you need some systematic way of identifying and grouping them. Possible ways of doing this are as follows:

1. Write the name of the theme in the margin of the text, for example 'compliance', and then actually cut up the transcripts so that you can group all the common

themes and categories. Before you get the scissors out, make sure that you have a photocopy of the whole transcripts, otherwise you may be in danger of taking things out of context.

2. Instead of cutting the transcripts up, try highlighting common themes with a highlighter pen. The problem with this is that the number of different concepts is limited to the number of different colours of your pens. Also, some concepts will belong to more than one theme.
3. Try transferring themes and concepts onto index cards, so that all common themes are located on the same card, but referenced to each subject.
4. Use a matrix to relate a number of key themes to different respondents. The results look a bit like a cross-tabulation, with cases or individuals down one side of the table and the main concepts running across the top. Individual cells can contain quotations.
5. Map the concepts and themes graphically using a cognitive map. Cognitive maps are similar to flow-charts that show how one theme or category influences another. Cognitive maps can be drawn up for each individual and summary maps can be developed. Cognitive maps are particularly useful in examining the process of personal decision-making.

For further information about using matrices and cognitive maps, read Miles and Huberman's *Qualitative Data Analysis* (1994). There are various software packages now available to assist you in this process and these are referenced at the end of this chapter.

Whichever method you go for, your overall aim is to identify the key concepts presented in the data. Once you have exhausted all the possible concepts you should start to find the same concepts reoccurring with different respondents. When you find differences between respondents, you should be looking for why those differences exist.

Eventually you may find links between some of the concepts, which in turn can be developed into common themes. At this point you may start moving away from just describing the data and instead start developing possible theories, which might help explain what you have found.

Remember when carrying out qualitative data analysis that it is an ongoing, dynamic process. You should come to the data with an open mind (although you need to acknowledge any biases that you think you may have) and thus the categories and themes that emerge from the data are not pre-set by you as the researcher. They should emerge from the data as issues and ideas, which are important and relevant to the respondents. One way of trying to validate your data analysis is to ask your respondents to look at your analysis of your interview with them and ask them if it is a true representation of what they said and believe.

For further details of how to analyse qualitative data, see Chapter 3, *Qualitative research*.

Coding open-ended questions

An open-ended question allows a respondent free reign to give any answer they want. Consequently, if we ask what we think is a very straightforward, open-ended question of 200 people, we could get back 200 different answers. This makes comparing the answers

Using interviews in a research project

very difficult. In fact, if we ask an open-ended question of lots of people we are likely to start building up some sort of pattern to the answers. We start to see some answers appearing more frequently than others. It is therefore possible to develop a coding frame to reflect the most frequently occurring and the most important answers to an open-ended question. The best way to do this is to examine a proportion of the answers you have received to a particular question and to use a five-bar gate system to record the most frequently cited answers. Once these have been established, each category can be assigned a nominal numerical value and all the answers given to the open-ended question can then be coded.

Exercise 3

In the following example we have listed all the answers given by a group of respondents to the following question:

'Why did you not take your medicine as the doctor requested you to?'
(Each one of these replies has been given by a different individual)
 I forgot.
 I didn't like the taste.
 I forgot.
 I was too busy.
 I left the bottle at home.
 I forgot.
 I got better and I didn't think that I needed it anymore.
 I forgot to take it that time.
 I was asleep.
 I forgot to take the antibiotics.
 I'd already eaten and I thought that I couldn't take it then.
 I was too busy.
 I forgot it.
 I was thinking of other things.
 I didn't feel ill any more.
 I felt better.
 I didn't need it.
 I never got it from the chemists.
 I just forgot.
 Forgot it.
 Forgot to take it.
 I don't remember what he told me to do.
 I felt better anyway.
 I forgot to take it.
 I was too busy.
 I was driving.
 I'd just eaten.
 I was at work.

1. Go through the replies listed above and try to identify those that are the most frequent. Draw up a coding frame to represent the main categories.
2. You may also want to pick up categories which are not very frequent, but which are very important.

Summary

In this chapter we have described:

- structured interviews
- semi-structured interviews
- unstructured/depth interviews.

You should by now be able to describe the advantages and disadvantages of the following methods:

- face-to-face interviews
- telephone interviews.

You should understand the difference between open-ended and closed questions and know what a pre-code is.

You should also be able to distinguish between a structured and a semi-structured interview. As you will recall, a structured interview with a majority of closed questions, with pre-coded answers, is appropriate when you are trying to directly compare the responses of a large number of people, whilst a semi-structured interview will allow you to ask more open-ended questions which are rich in detail but more difficult to analyse and compare.

You should be aware of the skills required to be a good interviewer and be able to list the ways in which interviewer error can be reduced.

You should be able to numerically code pre-coded and open-ended data collected in an interview.

Finally, you should be able to describe ways in which to analyse quantitative and qualitative data.

Answers to exercises

Exercise 1

There is no single right answer, however some possible suggestions are:

- train all the interviewers in the appropriate skills
- ensure that all the interviewers are thoroughly briefed on the research topic
- pilot the interview

Using interviews in a research project 133

- accompany interviewers and monitor their questioning and recording
- use structured questions where possible and avoid verbatim answers
- avoid having to select a pre-coded response from a verbatim answer – let the respondent select the code where possible
- avoid giving strong personal opinions, in particular do not show disapproval or disagreement with the respondent, regardless of what you may really think.

Exercise 2

1. Leading questions (by line number): 21, 23, 38, 41.
2. Ambiguous questions: 9, 38.
3. Two questions in one: 9, 14, 31, 50.
4. There is a danger that the interviewer could have confused or biased the interview. The interviewer assumes a number of things, for instance that the doctor was male, or that the chickenpox had made the child feel 'pretty ill'. Luckily the respondent actually corrects her on these points, but it may not always be so easy to pick up. If it's a minor matter, the respondent may not bother to clarify the question.
5. Questions should be phrased without assumptions, for example at line 21 the question 'You were worried about meningitis?' could be rephrased as 'What in particular were you worried about?'

    Likewise line 36 could be replaced with 'How important was that reassurance?'

    There are a number of questions where the interviewer asks two questions instead of one. The interviewer then has to probe the respondent's answer, otherwise she would not have been able to interpret the answer. Obviously it would be preferable to break up these multiple questions and ask them one at a time.

Exercise 3

1. Coding of open-ended questions is not an exact science and therefore two people coding the same group of answers are likely to produce slightly different coding frames. Nevertheless one would expect there to be some similarities. You could code the responses in the following way:

Forgot/did not remember	1
Got better/no longer ill/not needed	2
Too busy/thinking about other things	3
At work/left bottle at home	4
Eaten food so too late	5
Doing other things/driving/sleeping	6
Unpleasant taste	7
Did not take prescription to chemist	8

2. As you can see we have started off by coding the answers which produced the most frequent responses. We have also decided to combine some answers into a single

category. Note that although only one person said that they had not collected their prescription from the chemist, we have allocated this answer a separate code of its own since we felt that this was a particularly important answer. Likewise we have allocated a code for 'unpleasant taste', even though only one person said this.

References and further reading

Bell J (1995) *Doing your own Research Project*. Open University Press, Buckingham.

Carter Y and Thomas C (eds) (1997) *Research Methods in Primary Care*. Radcliffe Medical Press, Oxford.

Crombie I and Davies H (1996) *Research in Health Care*. John Wiley & Sons Ltd., Chichester.

King N (1994) The Qualitative Research Interview. In: C Cassell and G Simon (eds) *Qualitative Methods in Organisational Research*. Sage, London.

Mays N and Pope C (1995) Qualitative Interviews in Medical Research. *BMJ*. **311**: 251–53.

Miles M and Huberman A (1994) *Qualitative Data Analysis*. Sage, Thousand Oaks.

Moser C and Kalton G (1990) *Survey Methods in Social Investigation*. Gower, Hants.

Oakley A (1981) Interviewing Women: a contradiction in terms. In: H Roberts (ed) *Doing Feminist Research*. Routledge, London.

Oppenheim A (1992) *Questionnaire Design, Interviewing and Attitude Measurement*. Pinter Publishers Ltd., London.

Sapsford R and Jupp V (1996) *Data Collection and Analysis*. Sage, London.

Further resources

Software for qualitative data analysis

QSR Nudist is developed by: Qualitative Solutions & Research Pty Ltd., Box 171 La Trobe University Post Office, Victoria, Australia 3083. Email: nudist@qsr.latrobe.edu.au

Atlas-ti is developed by: Scientific Software Development, c/o Thomas Muhr, Tratenaustrasse 12, 10717 Berlin, Germany. Email: http://www.atlasti.de/

CHAPTER SIX

Data collection by observation

Nick Fox

Introduction

Imagine that you want to discover what goes on when elderly patients consult with a general practitioner or a practice nurse, or to find out how people utilise community pharmacists in their decisions about referral of symptoms to a GP, or to evaluate the skills of trainers in their educational activities with GP trainees. One way of researching these kinds of topics would be to interview those involved, or maybe even send out a questionnaire. From such methods, you could find out what the people involved thought about what was going on.

However, the best way to gain a 'rich picture' of a setting such as a surgery, a clinic or a pharmacy, is sometimes direct: by observation. Observational studies allow you – the researcher – to see for yourself what happens, rather than depending on your respondents.

Many studies of healthcare settings have used observational (or 'ethnographic') methods to explore what goes on, often in intimate interactions which happen behind closed doors. This chapter shows how we can use observation to enhance our understanding of these kinds of interaction, either as stand-alone descriptions or evaluations, or as part of research studies using a range of methods, including statistical analysis.

Having successfully completed the work in this chapter, including the exercises, you will be able to:

- describe what is involved in participant and non-participant observation, and the advantages of each approach
- give examples of the problems and pitfalls in carrying out observational research, based upon practical exercises
- produce guidelines for observation, note-taking, and writing up ethnographic data to maximise validity and reliability
- evaluate the ethical and philosophical issues in observational studies.

Working through this chapter

The study time involved in this chapter is approximately ten hours. In addition to the written text, the chapter includes exercises for completion. I suggest that as you work through the chapter, you establish for yourself a 'reflective log', linking the work in the chapter to your own research interests and needs, and documenting your reflections on the ethnographic method. Include your responses to the exercises plus your own thoughts as you read and consider the material.

Observation as a research method

Human beings spend much of their working life 'observing' the world in which they live. Perhaps it is evolutionarily advantageous to seek to know as much about our environment as we can, or maybe as a species, we are just curious! Either way, observing the world is something with which we are all familiar, even if we have never considered it as a way of carrying out formal research.

Immediately we should note that observation does not just involve vision: it includes all our senses, although in practice, sight and sound will be those which predominate in most research. And crucially, it also involves the *interpretation* of that sense data. No observer simply absorbs the visual or aural data that impinges on the sense organs: psychology has taught us that perception involves information processing, so that the pieces of data can be organised into something recognisable. Thus the light which falls on our retinas when we 'look' at a house causes nervous activity in the visual cortex of the brain. Based on experience, this activity leads to a perception, so that we see something that we recognise as 'house'.

This means that observation is more than just recording of data from the environment. When we observe, we are active collectors of data, not passive like a tape-recorder or video camera. Our brains are engaged as well as our eyes and ears, organising data so we can make sense of them. *Perception* is thus part of all human observation.

These aspects of observation are crucial to any efforts to use it as a method of research.

Exercise 1

Write down which kinds of factors may affect your perception of something you observe. You probably wrote down some of the following:

- factors associated with who you are, and your background
- your experiences of the situation, including whether you are familiar or not with what is happening
- your culture and how this interprets the situation you observe
- your attitudes and prejudices (some of which may be unconscious).

It follows from this that observation must be approached with some caution when it is to be adopted as a research method. In research we are not simply observing as part of human life, nor are we engaged in journalistic endeavours (which – however worthy – do not always aspire to the documentation of absolute 'truth'). Research is an activity which attempts to report aspects of the world in ways which minimise error and offer accounts which may be used for some purpose or another, for instance to improve patient care or to shape policy. To use the jargon of research methods, it seeks to be *valid* (accurate) and *reliable* (consistent).

This chapter outlines strategies for using observation in research so that the findings that emerge can be used with some confidence. It will introduce you to techniques of observation and help you develop both the skills to use observation and the understanding of the problems of validity and reliability. It will also acknowledge the criticisms of observation as a research method, which argue that it must remain subjective and 'unscientific'.

Of course, all empirical research uses observation in the sense that noting the readings on an instrument, or counting the bacteria in a microscope field are observations. This chapter, however, is concerned with a kind of social research, which is known as observational or ethnographic. Ethnography literally means 'writing culture'. It derives from anthropology and sociology, subjects which study other cultures and own cultures respectively. But all social settings are in this sense 'cultural', and as we shall see, ethnography or observation is often used where what we are trying to uncover are the norms, values, and shared meanings of those we are observing.

For example, in a GP surgery, ethnographic observation might consider the use of physical examinations. It would identify under what circumstances such examinations might be used, when within a consultation they occurred, and what strategies are used to ensure that they are conducted appropriately and in accordance with norms of modesty in the wider society. Thus the ethnographic study focuses on the culture of the GP surgery, perhaps considering the consequences for the effectiveness of the consultation, and when there may be problems.

Exercise 2

Consider the following ethnographic extract which describes an encounter on a surgical ward. What can you identify in the 'culture' of the encounter which may affect what is happening?

Fox N J (1992) *The Social Meaning of Surgery*
(*Mr D, the junior staff and the researcher gather round Patient Y's bed*)

Mr D	Hallo Mr Y. Well we want to send you home, but I don't like that raised temperature.
(*to patient, looking at chart*)	
Patient Y	No.
Mr D	I don't know what can be causing it. We've cultured the wound and there's no infection there. I just don't know what's causing it ... Are things ready for you to go home?

Patient Y	Yes, my wife can come and collect me today.
Mr D	Can you go to bed, and she can look after you?
Patient Y	Yes.
Mr D	I don't like that raised temperature. Phone your wife and you can go home now.
Patient Y	Thank you very much.

When and why should we use ethnographic methods?

To answer the question of when ethnography is an appropriate method, I would like you to read the following extract from Hammersley and Atkinson's *Ethnography: Principles in Practice* (1989: 6–7), which incidentally, is a good introductory text. Responding to traditional methods, which use a natural science perspective, they say:

> '... ethnographers have developed an alternative view of the proper nature of social research, often termed "naturalism" ... Naturalism proposes that, as far as possible, the social world should be studied in its "natural" state, undisturbed by the researcher. Hence "natural", not "artificial" settings like experiments or formal interviews, should be the primary source of data. Furthermore, the research should be carried out in ways that are sensitive to the nature of the setting. A key element of naturalism is the demand that the researcher adopt an attitude of "respect" or "appreciation" toward the social world. ... A first requirement of social research according to this view then, is fidelity to the phenomena under study, not to any particular set of methodological principles ... Moreover, social phenomena are regarded as quite distinct in character from natural phenomena ... the social world cannot be understood in terms of causal relationships or by the subsumption of social events under universal laws. This is because human actions are based upon, or infused by, social meanings: intentions, motives, attitudes, and beliefs. ... The same physical stimulus can mean different things to different people, and, indeed, to the same person at different times.
>
> ... According to naturalism, in order to understand people's behaviour we must use an approach that gives us access to the meanings that guide that behaviour. Fortunately the capacities we have developed as social actors can give us such access. As participant observers we can learn the culture or subculture of the people we are studying. We can come to interpret the world in the same way that they do.'

Later (1989: 23–4) they suggest that:

> 'The value of ethnography is perhaps most obvious in relationship to the development of theory. Its capacity to depict the activities and perspectives of actors ... challenge the dangerously misleading preconceptions that social scientists often

bring to research ... it is difficult for an ethnographer to maintain such preconceptions in the face of extended first-hand contact with the people and settings concerned. Furthermore, while the initial response to such contact may be their replacement by other misconceptions, over time the ethnographer has the opportunity to check his or her understanding of the phenomena under study. Equally importantly, though, the depiction of perspectives and activities in a setting allows one to begin to develop theory in a way that provides much more evidence of the plausibility of different lines of analysis than is available to the "armchair theorist", or even the survey researcher or experimentalist.

Also important here is the flexibility of ethnography. Since it does not entail extensive pre-fieldwork design, as social surveys and experiments generally do, the strategy and even the direction of the research can be changed relatively easily, in line with changing assessments of what is required by the process of theory construction.'

Exercise 3

Having read the above passages, answer the following self-assessment questions. According to Hammersley and Atkinson:

1. What should a naturalistic researcher attempt to achieve in his/her approach to research?
2. Upon what does the capacity of the ethnographer to interpret the phenomena s/he is studying depend?
3. Why is the theory developed by an ethnographer dependable (reliable)?

Exercise 4

Reflect on your recent work, and the setting in which you do that work. Think of something that has happened recently which you might research using this kind of observational or ethnographic method. What do you think your observational research would help you to explore or understand better?

At the end of this chapter, we will return to some of the issues which arise concerning the validity and reliability of ethnographic findings, but now we will turn to the practicalities of observational or ethnographic research. One of the first issues concerns the researcher's own position.

Observing in the field: finding a role

Have you ever been at a party or social gathering where you don't know many people? Apart from the few fortunates who are absolutely self-confident, this can be a daunting situation. How do you get started in social interactions with this bunch of people? And how do you avoid seeming like the stranger who knows nobody, and sticks out like a 'sore thumb'?

Ethnography – starting the collection of data in a field situation – can sometimes seem like this. The basic problem is deciding on a role for oneself. Of course you can wander round with a clipboard taking notes, but that could seem very intrusive and affect the setting you are trying to observe (it is against the spirit of 'naturalism' mentioned earlier).

One solution, which has been adopted by some researchers, is to become completely part of the field which one wants to research. The classic example is the study by Rosenhan (1973), in which sociologists managed to get themselves admitted as patients to a mental hospital. Once admitted, they openly took notes, yet because the staff were used to odd behaviour, did not think this unusual and indicative that the patients were not 'genuinely' ill. The sociologists gained in-depth knowledge of the hospital, including the experience of being an inmate. Another example of this kind of involvement was a study called *The World of Waiters* (Mars and Nicod 1984), which as the name implies was a study of the restaurant trade, in which the author took jobs as a waiter to carry out the research. Often, no-one will know that the researcher is other than a participant. This is known as *covert* research and raises ethical issues about the consent which people give before they become part of your research.

This kind of study might be called participant observation, in which the researcher has two roles – as observer and as participant. At the end of the last section I asked you to think about something which happened in your workplace, and how you might use observational research to study it. If you were to do so, you could adopt this kind of role, continuing in your work and at the same time acting as an observer.

Most of the time, however, it is not really feasible to become a participant. In my own research on surgery (1992), I could not work as a surgeon or a nurse, and did not fancy becoming a surgical patient! So I had to adopt a non-participant observer role, in which I took no part in the proceedings which I observed.

(N.B. Some authors do not accept this distinction, arguing that all observers participate to an extent. Hammersley and Atkinson (1989) distinguish a continuum between *complete participants* and *complete observers*.)

Exercise 5

Write down the advantages and disadvantages of participant and non-participant observation.

Exercise 6

To complete your reflections, write down some examples in healthcare which could best be studied by participant observers, and others where non-participant methods would be most appropriate. What are the factors that need to be considered in each case?

In summary, there are two principal methods of ethnographic study, the first taking on a dual role as both participant and observer, while in the second the researcher is only an observer. However, as noted earlier, there is a continuum between these positions. In some cases participants will be more overt in their observer role, and occasionally observers will start to participate (an example from my own experience of fieldwork was being asked to help out with menial tasks in the operating theatre when staff were short-handed). The latter may seem particularly appropriate where the setting is demanding and the researcher's help may be appreciated.

Becoming an observer

So far we have looked at the methodological differences between particular forms of observation. Now we look at the practicalities.

Exercise 7

To understand some of the problems and pitfalls of undertaking non-participant observation, I would like you to carry out the following exercise:

Undertake a 15-minute period of observation in a healthcare setting where you are not known personally. This setting could be a GP waiting room or out-patient clinic of a hospital, or a busy pharmacy, or a health and fitness club. You may need to use some ingenuity to gain access to this setting.

Either during, or immediately after this observation period, *make notes on what you observe(d)*. From your notes, write down some thoughts on what you feel are the interesting issues raised, both about the setting itself and about the process involved in gaining your data, using the de-briefing headings (*but don't look at these until you have completed the observation*).

(N.B. It would be advisable for you to take some means of identification with you when you go 'into the field'. Occasionally, the behaviour of an ethnographer can seem suspicious to others.)

Access

In the exercise that you just undertook, access might have been a big issue for you. If you were observing in a chemist's shop, you may have been able to pose as a customer, but if you tried this exercise in a GP waiting room without asking permission, I would have been surprised if someone had not queried your presence.

I intentionally did not raise the issue of gaining permission, leaving it to you to decide how to enter the field. So if you approached someone before doing your observation, you will already have experienced the need to be able to explain why you want to observe a setting. Hammersley and Atkinson (1989: 54) have this to say about gaining access:

> 'In many ways, gaining access is a thoroughly practical issue ... it involves drawing on the interpersonal resources and strategies that we all tend to develop in dealing with everyday life. But the process of achieving access is not merely a practical matter. Not only does its achievement depend upon theoretical understanding, often disguised as "native wit", but the discovery of obstacles to access, and perhaps

of effective means to overcoming them, themselves provide insights into the social organisation of the setting.'

Exercise 8

What issues are raised by this?

There are a number of points that I think are important here. Firstly, gaining access is not necessarily a single event: something once gained which is never again an issue. For example, you may have written a letter asking to observe a mother-and-baby clinic, and been given permission by the senior partner in a general practice. But when you arrive, you have to explain who you are and what you want to do. People may be surprised you do not have a questionnaire, and your presence may have to be explained to every patient at the clinic! So access is continuously negotiated throughout a period of fieldwork, and may be an issue until the moment you finish your observation.

Second, who do you approach to gain access? In the example of the clinic, it is highly unlikely that asking the GP surgery receptionist would be sufficient: imagine turning up at a clinic and telling the practice nurse or GP that it's all right for you to observe: their receptionist said so! Gaining adequate access requires you to know who has control of the setting and the power to grant access. This means that sometimes one finds oneself unintentionally complicit in the power relations of a setting, you are an imposition from above. For instance, if you are observing a hospital laundry, although you have management approval, the workers may not like the fact you have come to watch their work: you will be seen as a management spy. In such circumstances, the validity of your data may be compromised, as the workers will not behave 'naturally'.

(The classic example of this was a series of studies at the Hawthorne factory in the United States. Observers watched the production line workers in a bid to find ways to improve efficiency. After the study was analysed it was realised that the workers speeded up whenever they were observed, regardless of any other efforts to improve efficiency. This effect: the unintentional impact of observers on a setting, is now known as the 'Hawthorne Effect'.)

Thirdly, in some situations, access for observation cannot be obtained by asking permission. This may happen if those involved in a setting see their activities as sensitive in some ways, or because they feel insecure or threatened. Situations which entail intimate activities, such as physical examinations or disclosure of personal information, may be hard to observe. Settings which are normally closed to outsiders will also be hard to 'infiltrate'. For instance, the informal conversations among senior managers or among portering staff in a hospital will rarely be accessible, as these groups may not wish their private discussions to be overheard by an outsider. Legitimate issues of confidentiality may sometimes be used as a smokescreen by people (usually the powerful) who do not wish to be observed for one reason or another.

In such situations, we must once again consider covert observation, which may entail participant observation. Needless to say, it is probably a lot easier to become a porter than a senior manager. The ethics of such activity will be discussed later.

Methods of observation

We will look at the question of what you actually observe when you are an observer in the next section, but before that, it is worth thinking a little about the practicalities of observing.

Having gained access to a setting, the first thing to decide is when to do your observation, and it may not be immediately obvious without an initial foray into the field. For example, the daily activity of a GP surgery begins early in the morning. If you do not arrive until 11 am, much that may be relevant to a study will have been missed.

Secondly, you need to decide how often, and for how long, you will observe. These again cannot be legislated: you need to get into the field to find out what will be needed in order to gain an adequate picture. The time-scale must not be too short (I am sure you felt 15 minutes hardly gave any insight into the setting you observed) or too long: as with all research, observation is costly regarding your time and perhaps also those you observe. At some point you must decide you have sufficient data, and complete the observational phase of the research. I will return to this issue in 'Understanding and interpretation' on page 145.

Third, you need to find the right place to stand, and I mean this both physically and metaphorically. Physically, you need to be able to record what you observe, and this may mean negotiating a place, often in an unobtrusive position. For example, when observing ward rounds, I used to trail along at the back, and try to be as un-noticeable as possible. Metaphorically, you need to find a role for yourself which can be held consistently, and which you negotiate with those you observe so that they feel comfortable. This may mean explaining that you are not a management plant, and that you respect the confidentiality of some of what goes on. Often, saying that you are 'doing research' gives sufficient positioning for most people, and if you look the part, you will be thought of as a student! Such positioning is called 'filtering the presentation': giving everyone a version of yourself which will make them feel happy about your presence. (Note that this is also relevant in covert observation.)

At this point I want to raise an issue which you may have been wondering about. So far in this section, we have concentrated on *how* to observe – in other words with the practicalities. But the issue of how you observe raises the important question of *what* to observe. After all, who is to say that the GP surgery or pharmacy you chose can tell us anything about GP surgeries or pharmacies more generally? And perhaps the day you observed was quite atypical. So what generalisability is there to observation?

This is actually a huge issue, and perhaps you might like to re-read the extract from Hammersley and Atkinson on page 138, to start to get some answers. But I will return to this issue under the question of 'transferability' of research findings, in 'Validity and reliability in observational studies' on page 149.

Note-taking

What should be recorded from an observation session, and what should be left out? Your practical experience during the exercise will probably have raised this question immediately. In any setting one is faced with a myriad of events, and it is not possible, nor desirable, to note them all. So – as in real life – observational research has to be selective, and what you observe will largely depend upon the question you want to answer.

When you undertook the exercise in observation, you probably did not have an explicit research question, and often when one starts fieldwork it may be a general interest to document 'what goes on' that inspires researchers to adopt this methodology. But immediately you are faced with the complexities of a setting, you will form implicit interest areas.

Note-taking is of course essential. In most observational research notes will be handwritten, taken either at the time, or immediately afterwards. Sometimes it will be possible to use audio or video taping – for instance, to record a consultation between a GP and a patient for research or training purposes. However, such recordings will rarely stand alone as data, usually they will be transcribed or summarised in some way, and often it will be necessary for the researcher to add additional information to situate what has been recorded. For example, the audio record of what goes on in a GP reception area will provide accurate data on conversations, but may need the researcher's additional notes to pick up non-verbal detail, or the movements of people involved.

Taking notes may seem quite daunting because of the richness of a setting. To help to focus an ethnographer's attention, Spradley (1980: 78) suggests the following checklist of the kinds of things which could be recorded:

- space: the physical place or places
- actor: the people involved
- activity: a set of related acts people do
- object: the physical things which are present
- act: single actions that people do
- event: a set of related activities that people carry out
- time: the sequencing that takes place over time
- goal: the things people are trying to accomplish
- feelings: the emotions felt and expressed.

To this list I would add another point:

- reflection: your personal response to any of the above.

Exercise 9

Look back at your notes: how many of the above were part of your observation? You can probably remember some other things which fit these points that were not recorded in your notes: go back and try to flesh out your notes in these areas.

Finally, it is worth pointing out that your fieldnotes will not necessarily comprise just a record of what happened while you were observing. They may also include:

1. *Interview data.* These may be formal, or may comprise just snippets of interchanges, in which you ask someone to explain something or some event. For example, you may have watched a consultation between a GP and a patient. When the patient leaves, you may wish to ask the GP to clarify why s/he did something or asked a particular question. (I will talk more about the role of the 'key informant' below.)
2. *Documents.* Often in a field setting we come across relevant materials in the form of documents. These could be as wide-ranging as a poster on a GP surgery noticeboard or an official report or a letter. Often ethnographers will be shown such documents – it may take some negotiation to be able to take a copy of the original.
3. *Post hoc reflections.* Sometimes it is only when we have had some time to reflect on an observation session that we gain some insight, often when we are re-reading the notes or perhaps even in the middle of the night! Add these insights to the notes: they form a part of the continuing 'log' of your fieldwork.

Remember to date all entries in fieldnotes, including these *post hoc* insights.

Understanding and interpretation

I began this chapter with the comment that observation is not simply an act of the senses, it requires the brain to be engaged, to make sense of what we see or hear. Immediately we have observed something, our brains may start to work to interpret it. Let's take as an example the extract we looked at earlier:

Fox N J (1992) *The Social Meaning of Surgery*
(*Mr D, the junior staff and the researcher gather round Patient Y's bed*)

Mr D	Hallo Mr Y. Well we want to send you home, but I don't like that raised temperature.
(*to patient, looking at chart*)	
Patient Y	No.
Mr D	I don't know what can be causing it. We've cultured the wound and there's no infection there. I just don't know what's causing it ... Are things ready for you to go home?
Patient Y	Yes, my wife can come and collect me today.
Mr D	Can you go to bed, and she can look after you?
Patient Y	Yes.
Mr D	I don't like that raised temperature. Phone your wife and you can go home now.
Patient Y	Thank you very much.

What we have here is a brief piece of interaction. Having recorded this, we have to make some sense of it, if it is to be of any use as research data. Often the sense we make of something will depend upon our research commitments. Now for the sake of argument, let us imagine that what we are interested in is the information-seeking behaviour of surgeons.

We might pursue this objective by analysing how the surgeon here followed a checklist of questions to clarify what his decision (discharge or continuing hospital stay) should be. We would look at other examples, and see if this 'made sense'. If the surgeon followed a similar line of questioning, this proposition would be supported. If not, then we seek a new explanation.

If, on the other hand, the question concerned the different behaviours of surgeons towards male and female patients, we would interpret these data differently, perhaps picking up on the emphasis on the patient's marital status as a key.

How can we resolve this problem of multiple interpretation? Well, in some senses, there is no resolution, and we have to acknowledge that our understanding may be affected by all sorts of factors, not least what we are looking for.

One way to gain an understanding which is more valid and reliable is to try to find out what the surgeon and patient thought was happening, and it might be that to ask each in turn could elucidate more about the interaction. These kinds of 'triangulation' can help us be more certain that we are not interpreting things incorrectly.

The key informant

One very important person which features in many ethnographic studies is the 'key informant' (of course there may be a number of these). Finding a key informant can be a turning point in an observational study, because suddenly much of a setting can be explored through the eyes of one participant. One has to be cautious about the selection of the key informant, however, as their views are likely to be significant in shaping the explanatory framework and even the conclusions of your study. There is no such thing as a perfect key informant, but in general they may have one or more of the following characteristics (Hammersley and Atkinson 1989: 116–17):

- someone who, while part of the culture to be observed, is able to stand back – either by having come in from another culture, being new to the culture (the 'rookie'), having recently changed status, or someone whose nature is reflective or observant
- someone who likes and is willing to talk, either someone who is naïve and does not realise the import of her/his talk, or is frustrated or rebellious, or who is on the way out in terms of power once held but now forfeited, or who is a victim of power games in the setting
- someone who needs to talk to someone for their own emotional sustenance
- those with specialist knowledge.

Of these, those from category 1 may be the least involved, while those in categories 2 and 3 have strong investments which may colour their explanations, and whose words must therefore be carefully weighed. Those in category 4 will be valuable key informants, but may not disclose as much as the others.

In choosing a key informant, then, we need to weigh up what they are getting from the deal. No key informant's explanations can be given absolute privilege, and sometimes their accounts may need to be tested against others or against your observations to appraise their validity and reliability. For an interesting account of a study using a key informant, see Nigel Barley's entertaining ethnography of British customs, *Native Land*. Barley used a taxi driver as a key informant, often getting a very different slant on the customs he was exploring.

The whole question of understanding raises profound issues concerning the validity and objectivity of ethnography. We will return to this in the final part of this chapter.

Ethics of field work

I raised the issue of ethics earlier when discussing covert or participant research, but in all observational research there are a number of ethical issues which need to be addressed.

1. Confidentiality. One should take all possible measures to ensure that there are no consequences for those we observe as a result of subsequent identification in a report or published work. This means using pseudonyms, and if necessary ensuring that locations of research cannot be identified. Fieldnotes could contain much that could be seriously embarrassing to our subjects: they should be treated as confidential documents, and care should be taken to ensure they are not read by others.
2. Informed consent. People have a right to know that they are the subjects of research. If we take this as a principle, it raises issues about the use of any sort of covert observation, and of any intentional misinformation about the purpose of a piece of observation. It has been argued that this principle can be traded against the value of the findings of the research, either for those involved or for others.
3. Privacy. People have a right not to have their lives invaded. Once again this indicates problems with covert research, and the same trade-off arguments apply. However, we must be particularly careful to ensure that people do not feel an intrusion, however unintended (for example, by reading a research report and recognising themselves, however well-anonymised). It is well worth thinking about how to conduct observational research in an unobtrusive manner, to respect privacy of those who are being observed.
4. Validity of research. It is the view of some researchers that bad research is unethical. If your design is sloppy, and your findings of little value, then you have wasted everybody's time. The quality of a piece of research is an ethical issue in this sense, and we should attempt to conduct research in ways which maximise its validity.

Submissions to ethical committees

Ethical issues are notoriously slippery, and ultimately they will be argued and debated. However, it is important that the observational researcher acknowledges ethical issues, and that observers reflect upon what their research may mean for those involved. When it comes to healthcare research, ethical issues are particularly important where studies involve people who are already vulnerable as a consequence of illness. In such situations, many studies must go before an ethics committee, which is constituted from healthcare professionals, theologians and ethicists. They will take into account all the issues raised above.

Exercise 10

Although your earlier fieldwork study probably did not involve patients, imagine you are submitting a proposal to an ethics committee. Write down what you think were the ethical issues raised by the fieldwork exercise you undertook. Do you think you would have designed your observation differently in the light of this reflection? Address any questions which you think an ethics committee might have concerning this research.

Putting it into practice: the inside view

I hope that you have found these discussions of issues in fieldwork observation useful. To see what you have learnt, I want you to spend another period in practical observation, but with a slight difference.

Exercise 11

Choose a setting that you know well for this observation exercise. I recommend that you choose your own work environment. You can do this exercise either in your normal work time (which will give first-hand experience of the problems of playing a role and being an observer), or at a time when it is clear you are practising this observation and not working.

Do two specific things:

1. Find a key informant. Use the criteria suggested earlier in choosing someone. You will have to explain to this person what you are doing, just as you would in a real-life situation.
2. Ask your key informant to explain the use of spaces in the setting you have chosen. This is often the first thing that an ethnographer does when entering a setting, and may entail quite detailed mapping of the places involved. In particular, I want you to focus on what Goffman (1966) called 'front' and 'back' spaces. Front spaces are publicly accessible spaces, such as the general shop area in a pharmacy. Back spaces are only accessible by selected personnel, e.g. the staff in a pharmacy who are able to go behind the counter and into the dispensary. The interactions which go on in back spaces are often very interesting, and an observer needs to find out about these as part of his/her study of a setting.

Although you will probably know a lot about these spaces yourself, I want you to go through this with the informant, as it will give a focus for a fairly structured discussion.

Ensure you cover all the spaces, including those like coffee rooms or corridors, finding out what kinds of interactions go on in these spaces. Once you have gleaned this information, observe, either alone or with your informant, what really goes on in these spaces, looking for confirmations of what you had been told.

I suggest you allocate a maximum of one hour for this exercise, to include the time with the informant, and the observation. You may want to spend some additional time organising your notes from the observation and drawing maps of the front and back spaces.

In this chapter, we cannot go much further in terms of developing your fieldwork observation skills. I would certainly encourage you to read fieldwork guides and accounts of ethnographic studies, and some of these are given in the bibliography. However, practice is essential to develop these skills, and until you have to use observation in earnest, your skills may not really become more refined. If you wanted to practise, perhaps using the setting you have just explored, this would be valuable, and might even form a basis of a research study in due course!

However, I want now to turn to some further issues concerning the methodology of observation.

Validity and reliability in observational studies

The reliability and validity of a piece of research indicate its trustworthiness, in other words, the extent to which study findings reflect the world that we are seeking to explore in our observation. Reliability is concerned with the measuring tools we use in research, and whether they are consistent. Validity is an indicator of the accuracy of research – whether a study gives a true picture of what it is exploring. Reliability is a pre-requisite of validity, but does not guarantee it.

Validity and reliability are important issues for ethnographers – just as they are for all other researchers. However, because ethnography falls within a naturalistic and qualitative paradigm of research, we must think carefully about what validity and reliability mean for the way that we conduct observational studies. While the relevance of the trustworthiness of a piece of research still stands, Lincoln and Guba (1985) suggest that we can ask four key questions when designing or appraising qualitative research such as ethnography, and suggest terms to describe these issues:

1. How truthful is the finding? Credibility.
2. Can the findings be generalised? Transferability.
3. Could the findings be replicated? Dependability.
4. Can we rule out researcher bias? Confirmability.

These four questions relate to traditional (positivist) notions of study validity and reliability, as can be seen in the table below.

When carrying out observational research, we need to address the four issues of credibility, transferability, dependability and confirmability. However, Lincoln and Guba

Table 6.1 Positivist and naturalistic analyses of validity and reliability

Naturalistic	Positivist
Credibility *(Are the findings believable?)*	Internal validity
Transferability *(Are the findings applicable elsewhere?)*	External validity
Dependability *(If the study were repeated, would the same findings emerge?)*	Instrument reliability
Confirmability *(Has the researcher biased the findings?)*	Intra-observer reliability

(1985) argue that we need to think about some of these issues quite differently from the perspective of positivist research. Let us look at each area in turn.

Credibility

Related to the *internal validity* of a study, credibility requires that we concern ourselves with the accuracy of description in a piece of qualitative research. We need to state the precise parameters of the study – who was studied, where and when, and by what methods. If we identify these aspects, and if we have a reliable means of measurement (dependability and confirmability), our study will be valid for the specific setting investigated. We can add to the credibility of observations by using informants, who will ensure we are not misunderstanding what we observe. Use audio- or video-recording where possible to avoid inaccurate notes, and practice note-taking in field situations. Check out final reports with our informants too, to make sure inaccuracy has not occurred in analysis.

It is sometimes possible to use observation in conjunction with other methods, such as a survey. This can add to the credibility of findings, by 'triangulating': if findings from two sources agree, this supports the conclusions from each.

(Sometimes it is useful to use observation in the initial phase of research. Because of the richness of the data produced, it helps to focus the research on relevant issues, perhaps informing the construction of a questionnaire or interview schedule. Other programmes may begin with a survey to identify background factors and follow this with in-depth observation to flesh out the quantitative findings.)

Transferability

When de-briefing from the first observation exercise, I raised the question of whether it is possible to generalise from ethnographic data. After all, in most qualitative research, the method of sampling is not strictly representative, but will be aimed at maximising the diversity within the study setting, to ensure as 'rich' a picture of the setting as can be gleaned. Clearly, this method of sampling will not supply *external validity* in the way that is usually sought in quantitative research, which wishes to generalise beyond the study population.

Yet ethnographies often make claims that their findings are of value as more than just descriptions of a few isolated instances observed in a study. Part of the answer was raised in the Hammersley and Atkinson extract (see page 138): ethnography is a naturalistic method, which seeks to describe the world 'as it is' (the issue of credibility or internal validity discussed above). That, naturalistic researchers argue, is sufficient. In a major divergence from positivist approaches, Lincoln and Guba (1985) warn us that we must be very cautious when claiming transferability. In fact, they argue that no claims should be made about the applicability of the findings to other settings. If other researchers wish to generalise from a study to other situations, the onus must be on them rather than the original researcher to demonstrate a study's applicability elsewhere.

Dependability

The dependability of a study relates to the consistency of the measuring instrument, which in this case is the observer, and his/her capacity to make sense of the world. This 'instrument' should be able to draw the same conclusions from similar observations (internal reliability), while in theory, more than one observer should be in agreement when observing the same thing (inter-observer reliability). Note that dependability is essential (but not sufficient) to ensure credibility.

Positivist research (particularly in the natural sciences) assumes an unchanging world. To positivists, repeated studies, if identical, should produce identical findings. However, the naturalistic paradigm acknowledges that the social world is continually changing. Observational studies may themselves affect the world that they are attempting to measure, as with the previously mentioned Hawthorne studies. The presence of an observer, especially one who asks a lot of questions too, may lead subjects to reflect more fully on what – up to now – they took for granted.

If change is inevitable, dependability is a problem, because we cannot ensure that if we observe 'the same thing' on different occasions that it actually means 'the same thing' for the people involved. Lincoln and Guba (1985) suggest that in such a changing world, all an observer can do is to try to *predict* as much as possible of what these changes may be, and account for them by casting widely for data within the setting. Multiple examples are valuable because they give some evidence of continuity or consistency.

Confirmability

Confirmability could also be called objectivity or intra-observer reliability. It means that the instrument (the researcher) will not have an in-built bias such that some kinds of observation are treated differently from others.

However, in a naturalistic paradigm, we have to accept that observer bias is a fact of life: we all have values and we cannot wholly avoid allowing these to colour the way we interpret data in a qualitative analysis. To minimise this bias, ethnographers need to recognise their biases, and seek to fault their own assumptions or 'pet theories' about what they are researching. Informants are useful to remind an observer of his/her potential biases (although inevitably informants have biases too). Bringing in colleagues to offer alternative readings, and feeding back results of an analysis to the original respondents can help to reduce these biases. Again, you should be able to see how the confirmability of a study is a pre-requisite for its credibility.

Exercise 12

To ensure that you grasp these difficult discussions of validity and reliability, try to complete this exercise.

You want to conduct some observational research on the ways receptionists in a GP surgery deal with telephone requests for repeat prescriptions. What features of your research design do you build in to maximise credibility, transferability, dependability and confirmability?

Criticism of observational research

In this chapter, I have tried to provide an introduction to the practicalities of observational research, and addressed some of the theoretical issues which arise. All research methodologies have limitations, and each – be it a randomised controlled trial or an ethnography – is based on certain assumptions about the world which it seeks to explain or explore. There is certainly not time to go into the ramifications of the philosophy of science which have occupied natural and social scientists for centuries, but it is worth recognising that such debates exist and continue. I recommend readers to explore some of these debates if and when they have time, perhaps referring to a book such as Woolgar's *Science: The Very Idea* which offers an introduction in a concise format. For now, I want to merely point to two criticisms that have been levelled at ethnographic methods.

The first criticism is that ethnography, while useful for describing settings or situations, is compromised when it comes to trying to generate theoretical understanding which can help to explain more than just the specific instances observed. One recent proponent of this critique is Hammersley. He argues in *What's Wrong with Ethnography* (1992: 28) that:

> '... commitment to the goal of theoretical description on the part of ethnographers had led them to adopt what I call ... the reproduction model. From this point of view, ethnographic descriptions must simply portray the phenomenon of interest "in its own terms". However, this presumes that there is a single objective description of each phenomenon, and this is not the case: there are multiple, non-contradictory, true descriptions of any phenomenon. How we describe an object depends not just on decisions about what we believe to be true, but also on judgements about relevance. The latter rely, in turn, on the purposes which the description is to serve.

Much the same is true of explanations: what we take to explain a phenomenon depends not just on our ideas about what causes what, but also on the purposes for which the explanation is being developed. Ethnographers' commitment to the reproduction model obscures, from readers and perhaps even from ethnographers themselves, the relevances that structure their accounts. As a result, the rationales for those accounts may be incoherent; and wittingly or unwittingly, ethnography may become a vehicle for ideology.'

Hammersley's own commitment is to 'save' ethnography as a valid research tool, and he offers a resolution of his criticism later in his book, based on a 'critical realism' which attempts to recognise the possibility of interpretations which are valid. The work of Lincoln and Guba (1985) discussed earlier can also be seen as an effort to codify techniques of observation which will lead to consistent and accurate findings, while warning about generalisation. But for others, the value-laden character of interpretations based on observational studies mean that it cannot be considered as a scientific technique and must either be abandoned in favour of more rigorous methods, such as the survey or experiment, or limited to 'simple description'.

If this first criticism of ethnography is based on the multiplicity of possible explanations of observations, so too is the second. But this latter's concern is with the way in which observational studies (primarily in anthropology) have contributed to the construction – often aberrant or invidious – of identities for those who have been observed, while claiming objectivity for those doing the observing. This criticism has focused on the constructions of 'reality' in ethnographic accounts of field settings, and often has a political agenda in challenging the (superior) researcher's interpretation of the (inferior) subjects' lives. Crapanzano (1986: 51–2) writes that:

'Like translation, ethnography is also a somewhat provisional way of coming to terms with the foreignness of languages – of cultures and societies. The ethnographer does not, however, translate texts the way the translator does. He (sic) must first produce them. ... No text survives him other than his own. ... The ethnographer is a little like Hermes: a messenger who, given methodologies for uncovering the masked, the latent, the unconscious, may even obtain his message through stealth. He presents languages, cultures and societies in all their opacity, their foreignness, their meaninglessness; then like a magician, the hermeneut, Hermes himself clarifies the opaque, renders the foreign familiar, and gives meaning to the meaningless. He decodes the message. He interprets. ... The ethnographer does not recognize the provisional nature of his presentations. They are definitive. ... Embedded in interpretation, his presentations limit re-interpretation. Ethnography closes in on itself.'

Like others in this school of textual criticism of ethnography, Crapanzano questions this closing down that occurs in ethnographic texts such that the people represented become little more than ciphers in a code which the ethnographer has broken. They challenge the capacity of an ethnography to get at a single 'truth', and as with the first school of critics, point to the multiplicity of possible explanations of one's observations.

The consequences of this challenge are profound, and Tyler (1986: 123) suggests that observational studies must abandon explanation in favour of 'evocation': a mode of reflection which does not seek a truth, but rather tries to enable the observed's point of view to come across in reports of observations. This 'postmodern ethnography' de-privileges the author of an ethnographic report, and encourages a reflexivity in readers which can help them to sense something of the field setting and the people who are involved. It seeks to redress the imbalance between researcher and researched, giving the latter more of a voice than traditionally is the case in ethnography (as in almost all research).

I hope this brief exploration of some critiques of ethnography as a method has helped to point out that observational research must be conducted with one's eyes open. Not simply to what one observes, but also metaphorically, to the assumptions about how we try to know the world and give it meaning in the research process. I believe that these criticisms indicate a need for reflexivity on the part of anyone who wants to use observation in research – by which I mean a capacity to think about one's own part in creating the setting one is observing (both as a person there, and in the work of interpretation, which follows observation). In that spirit of reflexivity, I would invite you to complete this chapter in a final reflective exercise.

Exercise 13

1. What have you learnt concerning the uses of observation in research?
2. What do you think are the limitations of observational methods?
3. How might you respond to some of the criticisms of ethnography, both in how you behave 'in the field' and how you try to write up your interpretations?
4. Why do those who use observational methods in research need to be 'reflexive'?

Conclusion

Observation is a well-established methodology for exploring the social world, and should be considered in situations where detailed descriptions of a setting and the meanings and values of its inhabitants need to be explored. Observation needs to be approached in a rigorous and structured way, both in terms of the techniques used to gather data, and the methodological considerations of validity, reliability and the ethics of research. Some criticisms of ethnography challenge the possibility to provide accurate explanations of settings, and researchers need to be reflexive about their own activities as researchers and writers of observational studies.

Answers to exercises

Some of the exercises in this chapter are to a large extent based on self-selected examples. It is not feasible to provide specific answers for these, but you should draw on the guidelines provided in the text when approaching them.

Exercise 2

You may have written down:

- the ceremonial form of the 'ward round' with consultant and junior staff
- the physical arrangements of the surgical ward, including the relative position of the patient (lying down) and surgeon (standing)
- the recourse to technical knowledge of pathology
- the use of the chart as a datum accessible and comprehensible only to the staff
- the dependency of the post-operative patient
- the marital arrangements of the patient and the cultural assumptions implicit in the questions asked about these.

You may have others too – there is potentially great richness in such a short extract.

So, when we use the term ethnography to describe the method of observation, we are reminded that what goes on is not always simply a 'rational' activity, but has a richness associated with the meanings which such activities have for participants. And it is because observation can get at such meanings – some would argue in a way that none other can (Geertz 1983) – that it is a useful method for use when researching health and healthcare.

Exercise 3

1. The ethnographer attempts to study phenomena in their natural setting and to acknowledge or 'respect' the characteristics of that setting. S/he sets out to understand the meanings of phenomena occurring in the settings for the people who are involved, and as far as possible to avoid preconceptions.
2. Hammersley and Atkinson argue that because we are ourselves part of the social world (we are 'social actors') then we understand much about the rules of social life and can apply this to what we observe during ethnographic research.
3. They argue that the theory that is developed in an ethnographic study is based on first-hand experience in the field rather than from the comfort of an armchair. Secondly, it is not affected by an artificial research design (as happens in surveys and experiments). Finally, because ethnography involves extended contact, there is much more evidence upon which to base theory, and the researcher's biases are likely to be attenuated over time, making these data reliable (dependable).

In summary, we can see from this that observation is valuable where we can access natural settings, where we are interested in the meanings which people give to phenomena in those settings, and where we may want to develop theoretical understanding of what is going on. For instance, a researcher may want to know what happens when people from non-British backgrounds consult with a GP. This research is best carried out in the actual setting of the GP consultation. It depends on understanding the perspectives, attitudes and values of the participants, and we want to move from the raw findings to a theory of what is happening – perhaps focusing on language difficulties or cultural differences.

Exercise 5

1. The advantages of participant observation mainly derive from the fact that the researcher's presence is unlikely to affect the setting, because her/his presence as researcher is masked by the role of participant. But this is a disadvantage too, because the roles are confused, and it is quite possible that the participant role will bias the way the observer perceives what is going on. Another disadvantage is that the observer may miss vital things because s/he is too busy participating. Covert research may not be considered ethical and there are issues about deceiving subjects and their rights to privacy.
2. Non-participant observation has the advantage of being unbiased, but the disadvantage of potentially affecting the interactions. It has the advantage of enabling detailed observations to be made without distraction, but there may be a problem with gaining access – with some aspects of a setting being 'off-limits' to an outsider, or subjects refusing to be observed. There is also the problem mentioned at the start of this section, of finding a way of being unobtrusive even though the researcher does not seem to have a role within the setting. Non-participant observation has the advantage that it can be applied in many more settings, as the researcher does not need to become 'part of the action'.

Exercise 6

It is difficult to provide any guideline answer.

Exercise 7

If you found this a challenging experience, then you are in good company: almost every ethnographer finds the first entry into 'the field' daunting, and difficult, especially if it is unfamiliar territory. You may have felt uncomfortable, visible and vulnerable. Coping with these feelings is an important issue, because they can be so dominant that it becomes impossible to observe anything at all!

Write down your reflections under the following headings.

Main themes
What are the themes that your notes indicate are of importance for understanding this setting? These may take the form of very tentative ideas or questions that further observation or interviews might elucidate.

Access
How did you choose the setting? How did you negotiate access? How did you explain your presence to anyone who asked? How did you sustain your presence as an outsider in this setting? What could you do differently to enhance access? Do you think your presence may have affected what went on?

Method of observation
What procedures did you use to organise your observations? Was the time frame (15 minutes) appropriate, and if not, how might you decide how long is needed? Were you able to find a suitable place from which to conduct your observations? What might you do differently next time?

Note-taking
How did you take notes? Were you able to take notes during the observation? What did you take notes about, and how did you choose what to report? How accurate do you think your notes are? And how could you improve their accuracy?

Understanding
How did you make sense of what you observed? Were there any incidents which you could not understand? How would you go about getting the views of a participant on areas which you do not understand?

Ethics
What do you think were the ethical issues involved in your undertaking this observation as a non-participant? How do you balance these against the opportunities which observation gives to obtain accurate data about a setting?

Make a list of any other issues not addressed in these headings.

Exercise 11

I hope you found this an interesting experience, particularly because it required formal observation of a setting you know very well. Did you glean any new insights about this environment? What were the consequences of choosing a setting in which you are perhaps a regular participant? Use the headings that we used earlier to de-brief from this exercise:

Main themes
What are the themes that your notes indicate are of importance for understanding this setting? These may take the form of very tentative ideas or questions that further observation or interviews might elucidate.

Access
How did you choose the setting? How did you negotiate access? How did you explain your presence to anyone who asked? How did you sustain your presence as an outsider in this setting? What could you do differently to enhance access? Do you think your presence may have affected what went on?

Method of observation
What procedures did you use to organise your observations? Was the time frame (one hour) appropriate, and if not, how might you decide how long is needed? Were you able

to find a suitable place from which to conduct your observations? What might you do differently next time?

Note-taking

How did you take notes? Were you able to take notes during the observation? What did you take notes about, and how did you choose what to report? How accurate do you think your notes are? And how could you improve their accuracy?

Understanding

How did you make sense of what you observed? Were there any incidents that you could not understand? How would you go about getting the views of a participant on areas that you do not understand?

Ethics

What do you think were the ethical issues involved in your undertaking this observation as a non-participant? How do you balance these against the opportunities which observation gives to obtain accurate data about a setting?

Exercise 12

Credibility

What you need to do is try to ensure that your description is accurate. Negotiate good access, and make sure you can observe what is going on (this may entail a means of listening in to telephone conversations. Practice note-taking, and use audio-tape for interviews, and perhaps to record the conversations. Make sure you document precisely all features of the setting (perhaps starting with the spaces, as in the practical exercise), who was observed, and when. Talk to those people involved (the receptionists) to find out what they think they are doing, and when you draw conclusions, feed these back to the participants to see if they agree with your findings.

Transferability

You do not make claims about the generalisability of the study, but by documenting the parameters (who, when, where) other researchers or policy-makers can judge the limits of transferability to other settings.

Dependability

To try to recognise the variability in the setting, and its changing character, you try to account for this variability: documenting different instances and situations and the different personnel involved (not just one or two receptionists). In this way, try to describe the setting as fully as possible. If you think there may be changes occurring (even perhaps as a result of your observation) leave the field and return later, making observations on different days. *In extremis*, consider the possibility of covert observation (recording telephone calls without receptionists' knowledge).

Confirmability

To try to avoid biases (for example, drawing conclusions based on personal experience) you try to reflect on what those biases might be and check with informants that you are not making incorrect assumptions. When it comes to analysing data, ask friends or colleagues to read your interpretations and come up with queries or alternative explanations.

I hope you identified some of these aspects of how to maximise the validity and reliability of this study. Appraising validity and reliability are essential for research to be worthwhile, and any observational research design needs to think about these four aspects before entering the field. Bear in mind the earlier argument that bad research is not only a waste of time but also unethical.

References

Barley N (1990) *Native Land*. Penguin Books Ltd, London.

Crapanzano V (1986) Hermes' dilemma: the masking of subversion in ethnographic descriptions. In: J Clifford and G E Marcus (eds) *Writing Culture*. University of California Press, Berkeley.

Fox N J (1992) *The Social Meaning of Surgery*. Open University Press, Buckingham.

Geertz C (1983) *Local Knowledge*. Basic Books, New York.

Goffman E (1966) *Behaviour in Public Places: Notes on the Social Organization of Gatherings*. Prentice Hall, New York.

Hammersley M (1992) *What's Wrong with Ethnography*. Routledge, London.

Hammersley M and Atkinson P (1989) *Ethnography. Principles in Practice*. Routledge, London.

Lincoln and Guba (1985) *Naturalistic Inquiry*. Sage, California.

Mars G and Nicod M (1984) *The World of Waiters*. Allen & Unwin, London.

Rosenhan D L (1973) On Being Sane in Insane Places. *Science*. **179**: 250–58.

Spradley J P (1980) *Participant Observation*. Holt, Rinehart and Winston, New York.

Tyler S (1986) Postmodern ethnography: from document of the occult to occult document. In: J Clifford and G E Marcus (eds) *Writing Culture*. University of California Press, Berkeley.

Further reading

Clifford J and Marcus G E (eds) (1986) *Writing Culture*. University of California Press, Berkeley.

Hammersley M (1992) *What's Wrong with Ethnography*. Routledge, London.

Hammersley M and Atkinson P (1989) *Ethnography. Principles in Practice*. Routledge, London.

Woolgar S (1988) *Science: The Very Idea*. Ellis Horwood, Chichester.

Glossary

Action research — interventions in real-life situations involving practitioners, e.g. introducing a specialist practitioner role in the practice setting.

Anonymity — is the protection of the identity of research subjects such that even the researcher cannot identify the respondent to a questionnaire. Questionnaires in an anonymous survey do not have an identification number and cannot be linked back to an individual. (Anonymity should not be confused with confidentiality, where individuals can be identified by the researcher.)

Association — between two variables represents some sort of relationship. An association can be a causal one or it might be spurious. Associations can be positive or negative.

Bias — is a derivation of the results from the truth. This can either be due to random error or, more likely, due to systematic error. The latter could be caused by, for example, sampling or poor questionnaire design.

Case — is a unit of analysis. Usually this takes the form of an individual subject but it could be a different unit of analysis altogether, such as a family or a blood culture.

Case studies — an in-depth study of a single or small number of units. The unit may be individual people, patients, groups or organisations, e.g. evaluating a new service.

Categorical data — see *Nominal data*.

Closed question — is one where the possible answers have been defined in advance and so the respondents' answers will be restricted to pre-coded responses offered. A pilot study should be carried out to decide on the correct pre-codes.

Cluster sampling — is used when the population is diversely spread over a geographical area and for various reasons it is preferable to use groups of subjects from several sites rather than randomly selecting the whole sample from the whole population, e.g. to investigate the grades of community nurses employed nationally the sample could select a sample of community nurses in one NHS trust in each of the health regions.

Coding is the process by which responses to questionnaires or other data are assigned a numerical value or code in order that the data can be transferred to a computer for data analysis. (See also *pre-codes, closed questions, open-ended questions* and *re-coding*.)

Cohort design is a longitudinal design where the same individuals are interviewed or observed repeatedly over time. Respondents usually share a common characteristic.

Concept is an abstract idea or mental construct representing some event or object in reality.

Confidentiality is the protection of the identity of research subjects so that identities cannot be revealed in the research findings and the only person who can link a respondent's completed questionnaire to a name and address is the researcher. A questionnaire with just a coded identification number is confidential. (This should not be confused with anonymity, where not even the researcher can identify the subjects.)

Confounding variable is one which systematically varies with the independent variable and also has causal effect on the dependent variable. The influence of a confounding variable may be difficult to identify, since it is sometimes difficult to separate out the independent variable from any confounding variables in real life.

Constant error can be caused by the presence of a confounding variable in an experiment. It is also an alternative term for systematic bias.

Construct validity is the extent to which the measurement corresponds to the theoretical concepts (constructs) concerning the object of the study. There are two kinds of construct validity: convergent and divergent.

Content analysis is the systematic examination of text or conversational transcripts to identify and group common themes, and to develop categories for analysis.

Content validity is a set of operations or measures that together operationalise all aspects of a concept.

Convenience	is also called incidental sampling. Utilises readily available subjects and sampling often used in small-scale, localised research projects. The sample may not be representative of the population as a whole and the results may not be generalisable, e.g. patients selected from one geographical area, such as an electoral ward, may have particularly high or low levels of deprivation.
Correlation studies	investigations into the relationship between two variables, but interested in identifying associations rather than cause and effect, e.g. is there a relationship between social group and the number of GP consultations?
Criterion validity	is the extent to which measurement correlates with an external indicator of the phenomenon. There are two types of criterion validity – concurrent and predictive. Concurrent validity is a comparison against another external measurement at the same point in time. Predictive validity is the extent to which the measurement can act as a predictor of the criterion. Predictive validity can be useful in relation to health since it can act as an early risk indicator before a condition develops in full.
Cross-sectional design	is analogous to a snapshot. A cross-sectional design is one which focuses on a single, fixed period in time, and can provide a description of respondents that differ on a number of variables.
Delphi technique	is a method for obtaining expert or consensus opinion on a particular topic, by using multiple 'rounds' or waves of questions whereby the results from the previous rounds are continually fed back to the same respondents to bring about a group consensus.
Dependent variable	is known as the outcome variable. The value of a dependent variable is dependent on other independent variables and its value will change as the independent variable or intervention changes. Statistical techniques can be used to predict the value of the dependent variable. An example of a dependent variable might be peak flow or blood pressure.
Descriptive design	is one which seeks to describe the distribution of variables for a particular topic. Descriptive studies can be quantitative, for instance a survey, but they do not involve the use of a deliberate intervention. However, it is possible to

	carry out correlational analysis of the existing variables in a descriptive study.
Descriptive statistics	are used to describe and summarise variables within a data set, including describing relationships between variables. They do not seek to generalise the findings from the sample to the wider population, unlike inferential statistics.
Error	can be due to two sources: random error and systematic error. Random error is due to chance, whilst systematic error is due to an identifiable source, such as sampling bias or response bias.
Ethnography	qualitative investigation of cultures and population subgroups which seeks to explore, describe and explain cultural behaviour, e.g. understanding of mental illness within a particular Asian subgroup.
Experimental design	controlled investigations which try to establish cause-and-designs effect between two or more variables with the purpose of predicting outcomes, e.g. whether one type of medication is more effective than another in treating a particular illness.
External validity	relates to the extent to which the findings from a study can be generalised (from the sample) to a wider population (and be claimed to be representative).
Extraneous variable	is a variable other than the independent variable which may have some influence on the dependent variable and may be a potential confounding variable if it is not controlled for.
Face validity	is the extent that the measure or instrument being used appears to measure what it is supposed to, e.g. a thermometer might be said to possess face validity.
Focus groups	is a method of collecting qualitative data from a group of people. It takes the form of a group discussion, ideally with 6–8 respondents. A moderator directs the group discussion.
Grounded theory	is a technique for analysing qualitative data and generating concepts and theories, inductively, using a constant comparative method.
Hawthorne effect	is the changes that occur in a subject's behaviour or attitude as a result of being included in the study and

being placed under observation. (The term derives from industrial psychological studies that were carried out at the Hawthorne plant of the Western Electric Corporation in Illinois in the 1920s and were reported by Mayo. He found that whatever experimental environmental conditions were tried out on the workers, productivity always went up. He realised that it was the effect of actually being under study that resulted in a change of behaviour and so increased productivity.)

Hypothesis is a statement about the relationship between the dependent and the independent variables to be studied. Traditionally the null hypothesis is assumed to be correct, until research demonstrates that the null hypothesis is incorrect. (See *Null hypothesis*.)

Incidence can be defined as the number of new spells of a phenomenon, e.g. illness, in a defined population in a specified period. An incidence rate would be the rate at which new cases of the phenomena occur in a given population. (See *Prevalence*.)

Incidental sampling see *Convenience sampling*.

Independent variable is one which 'causes' the dependent variable. The independent variable takes the form of the intervention or treatment in an experiment and is manipulated to demonstrate change in the dependent variable.

In-depth interview takes an unstructured, qualitative approach. The questions asked will be mostly open-ended and overall the degree of control over both the order and content of the interview is less than in a structured interview.

Indexing is a process of collating indicators to create a single index of a particular phenomenon such as mental health, quality of life, daily functioning, etc.

Indicator is the operationalised form of a concept. In research, concepts need to be tightly defined so that they can be measured. To measure a concept we have to translate it into a specific indicator.

Instrument validity is the extent to which the instrument or indicator measures what it purports to measure. (Note that a study could have instrument validity but still lack validity overall due to lack of external validity.)

Internal validity	relates to the validity of the study itself, including both the design and the instruments used.
Interval data	is measured on an interval scale where the distance between each value is equal and the distance between values is the same anywhere on the scale. Interval level data does not possess a true zero, unlike ratio-level data.
Intervening variable	occurs in the causal pathway between the independent variable and the dependent variable. It is statistically associated with both the independent and the dependent variable.
Intervention	is the independent variable in an experimental design. An intervention could take the form of treatment, such as drug treatment. Those subjects selected to receive the intervention in an experiment are placed in the 'intervention' group.
Interview schedule	is a list of questions used in an interview.
Longitudinal study	is one in which groups of people are interviewed repeatedly over a period of time. A cohort study is where the same group of people are followed up over time. However, if a group of different people are interviewed in each wave of a survey this is known as a trend design.
Mean	is a measure of central tendency. It is calculated by summing all the individual values and dividing this figure by the total number of individual cases to produce a mean average. It is a descriptive statistic which can only be applied to interval data.
Median	is a measure of central tendency. It is the mid-point or middle value where all the values are placed in order. It is less susceptible to distortion by extreme values than the mean, and is a suitable descriptive statistic for both ordinal and interval data.
Mode	is a measure of central tendency. It is the most frequently occurring or most common value in a set of observations. It can be used for any measurement level but is most suited for describing nominal or categorical data.
Nominal data	also known as categorical data, is a set of unordered categories. Each category is represented by a different numerical code, but the codes or numbers are allocated on

an arbitrary basis and have no numerical meaning. (See also *Ordinal data* and *Interval data*.)

Null hypothesis is the alternative hypothesis. It usually assumes that there is no relationship between the dependent and independent variables. The null hypothesis is assumed to be correct, until research demonstrates that it is incorrect. This process is known as 'falsification'.

Open-ended question is one which allows the respondent the freedom to give their own answer to a question, rather than forcing them to select one from a limited choice. Open-ended questions are commonly used in in-depth interviews, but they can also be used in quantitative structured interviews as well.

Ordinal data is composed of a set of categories which can be placed in an order. Each category is represented by a numeric code which in turn represents the same order as the data. However, the numbers do not represent the distance between each category. For instance, a variable describing patient satisfaction may be coded as follows: Dissatisfied 1, Neither 2, Satisfied 3. The code 2 cannot be interpreted as being twice that of code 1.

Panel study is another term for a longitudinal or cohort study, where individuals are interviewed repeatedly over a period of time.

Phenomenology descriptions of individuals' lived experience of events, e.g. the experience of caring for someone with pre-senile dementia.

Population is a term used in research which refers to *all* the potential subjects or units of interest who share the same characteristics which would make them eligible for entry into a study. (See *Sampling frame*.)

Prevalence is the number of cases as subjects with a given condition or disease within a specified time period. The prevalence of a condition would include all those people with the condition, even if the condition started prior to the start of the specified time period. (See also *Incidence*.)

Prospective study is one that is planned from the beginning and takes a forward-looking approach. Subjects are followed over time and interventions can be introduced as appropriate.

Purposive sampling	subjects are selected because they have special knowledge of the topic under investigation, e.g. key stakeholders in an organisation.
Qualitative research	deals with the human experience and is based on analysis of words rather than numbers. Qualitative research methods seek to explore rich information usually collected from fairly small samples and include methods such as in-depth interviews, focus groups, action research and ethnographic studies.
Quantitative research	is essentially concerned with numerical measurement and numerical data. All experimental research is based on a quantitative approach. Quantitative research tends to be based on larger sample sizes in order to produce results which can be generalised to a wider population.
Questionnaire	is a set of questions used to collect data. Questionnaires can be administered face-to-face by an interviewer, over a telephone or by self-completion. Questionnaires can include closed and open-ended questions.
Quota sample	is a form of non-random sampling and one that is commonly used in market research. The sample is designed to meet certain quotas, set usually to obtain certain numbers by age, sex and social class. The sample selected within each quota is selected by convenience, rather than by random methods.
Random error	is non-systematic bias which can negate the influence of the independent variable. Reliability is affected by random error.
Randomisation	is the random assignment of subjects to intervention and control groups. Randomisation is a way of ensuring that chance dictates who receives which treatment. In this way all extraneous variables should be controlled for. Random allocation does not mean haphazard allocation.
Randomised control trial (RCT)	is seen as the 'gold standard' of experimental design. As the name implies, subjects are randomly allocated to either the intervention or the control group.
Ratio-level data	is similar to interval data in that there is an equal distance between each value, except that ratio-level data does possess a true zero. An example of ratio-level data would be age.

Glossary

Re-coding — is the process of altering the codes assigned to a particular variable, usually by aggregating categories. For instance, continuous interval data such as age may be re-coded into age bands, thus making it ordinal data. Re-coding allows data to be analysed and compared in different ways than in its original state.

Reliability — a term which refers to the ability of the data collection tool to give consistent results, e.g. a 12-inch ruler would consistently measure an item as being the same length irrespective of how many times it was used or who used it.

Representativeness — is the extent to which a sample of subjects is representative of the wider population. If a sample is not representative, then the findings may not be generalisable.

Respondent — the people who agree to take part in a research project and from whom data are collected.

Response rate — is the proportion of people who have participated in a study or completed a question. It is calculated by dividing the total number of people who have participated by those who were approached or asked to participate.

Retrospective design — is one which looks backwards over time, often using data already collected by others. It usually takes the form of correlational research, identifying relationships between independent and dependent variables.

Sample — is a group or subset of the chosen population. A sample can be selected by random or non-random methods. Findings from a representative sample can be generalised to the wider population.

Sampling — the selection of subjects from the population under study.

Sampling frame — is the pool of potential subjects which share a similar criteria for entry in to a study. (See also *Population*.)

Sequential sampling — the size of the sample is not preset. The researcher collects data from each subject in turn until s/he is satisfied that there is no new information for collection – the topic is saturated. Used mostly in qualitative research, e.g. in setting up a new service, potential users of the service are asked what they would want until no new ideas emerge.

Snowballing — is a non-probability method of sampling commonly employed in qualitative research. Recruited subjects nominate other potential subjects for inclusion in the study.

SPSS	(Statistical Package for the Social Sciences) is an increasingly popular and easy-to-use software package for data analysis.
Stratified sampling	is used when the population contains subgroups and it is necessary to ensure that representatives of all groups are included, e.g. patients in different age bands, nurses employed on different professional grades, healthcare staff from a range of professions. Randomisation within each subgroup can be applied.
Survey	is a method of collecting large-scale quantitative data, but does not use an experimental design. With a survey there is no control over who receives the intervention or when. Instead, a survey design can examine the real world and describe existing relationships. A survey can be either simply descriptive or a correlation.
Systematic sampling	involves taking the *n*th name on a list, such as every third person or every tenth. Sometimes used by researchers who claim to have used random sampling, but factually this approach automatically eliminates certain members of the population who may have a perspective which is useful to the study but goes unnoticed, e.g. taking the first-named member of the household from an electoral poll will almost certainly eliminate the younger members of the population.
Theoretical sampling	is a sampling method used in qualitative research, whereby the sample is selected on the basis of the theory and the needs of the emerging theory. It does not seek to be representative.
Validity	is the extent to which a study measures what it purports to measure. There are many different types of validity.
Variable	is an operationalised concept. A variable is a phenomenon that varies and must be measurable. An outcome variable is known as the dependent variable and the effect variable is known as the independent variable. The independent variable has a causal effect on the dependent variable.
Weighting	is a correction factor which is applied to data in the analysis phase to make the sample representative. For instance, if a disproportionate stratified sampling technique has been used, then the total data may need to be

re-weighted to make them representative of the total population. Weighting is also used to correct for non-response, when the respondents are known to be biased in a systematic way.

Index

access 16, 141–2
accuracy
    observational studies 150
    sample size 89
action research 10
aim 5
anonymous survey 104
artefacts 65–6
associations 9, 45
attitudinal information 115
attrition 79

baseline 30, 37, 41
between-subject designs 39–40
bias 14, 67
    interviews 120–1, 123
    observation 152
    systematic 39
body language 125

case studies 10, 61
categories 69, 73–4
causality 45
census 78
closed questions 12, 92
cluster sampling 15, 86–7
coding 68–9, 94–5, 130–1
cognitive maps 130
cohort surveys 78–9
communication skills 113, 123
community trials 43
computers, data analysis 18, 72–3
conclusions 18–19
confidence interval 89
confidential survey 104
confidentiality 147
confirmability 149, 151–2
confounding variables 30, 38
constant comparative analysis 60, 67
content analysis 69–71, 94
content validity 29
context, interviews 113
contingency tables 105, 129
control groups 9, 30–2

convenience sampling 15, 87
correlation studies 9, 58
correlational surveys 79
covering letter 103
covert research 140
credibility 149, 150
critical realism 153
cross-over design 38
cross-sectional surveys 78
cross-tabulations 105, 129
cues 115, 125
culture 137–8

data
    see also measurement; sampling
    analysis 17–18, 68–73, 105–6, 128–32
    coding 94–5
    collection 11–14, 17, 60, 62–6, 81–4
    computerised analysis 18, 72–3
    handling 66–8
    quality 113
    recording 125
dependability 149, 151
dependent variables 24, 42
depth interviews 63–4
disproportionate sampling 86
documentation 66
drop-outs 39

efficiency, surveys 79–80
empathy 124
error
    interviews 120–1
    systematic 28
ethical issues 16, 46–7
    interviews 123
    observation 147–8
ethnography 10, 59, 137–41
evidence, hierarchy of 44–5
evocation 154
experimental designs 9, 23–53
explanatory surveys 79

external validity 45–6
   surveys 79
extraneous variables 30

face-to-face interviews 115–16
face-to-face surveys 81
factorial designs 43
fatigue 39
filtering 119
Flesch Reading Ease Score 96, 103
flexibility, surveys 80
focus groups 64, 116–17
focused interviews 63
Fog Index 96, 103, 111
frequencies 129

generalisability 61
grounded theory 11, 59–60
group interviews 64, 116–17

Hawthorne effect 33, 142
hierarchy of evidence 44–5
hypothesis 5, 25–6

identifier 91–2
in-depth interviews 63–4, 115, 126
incidental sampling 15
independent variables 24, 27, 43
indexing data 69
indices, questionnaires 101
information 34–5
   attitudinal 115
informed consent 34, 46
   interviews 119–20
   observation 147
internal validity 45–6, 79, 150
interpretation 136, 145–8
interpretation error 121
interrogation error 121
interval data 96
intervention 27
intervention group 9
interviews 11–12, 13, 60, 63–4
   bias 120–1, 123
   data analysis 128–32
   respondents 119–20
   schedule 121–3
   techniques 123–6
   training 113, 118, 123
   transcription 66–8
   types 63–4, 114–18
investigation 3

key informant 146–7

leading questions 122
Likert scale 99–100
listening skills 123
literacy 91
literature review 6–7
longitudinal surveys 78–9

manifest level 69
matched-pair designs 40–1
matrices 130
maturation 38
mean 97
measurement
   potency 29–30
   reliability 27–8
   validity 28–9
median 97
medical jargon 122
methodology 7–19
multiple examples 151
multiple interpretation 146

negative reinforcement 123
nominal data 94–5
non-participant observation 140
non-random sampling 87–8
non-verbal cues 125
note-taking 144–5
null hypothesis 26

objectivity 151
observation 12, 14, 135–59
   see also ethnography
   access 141–2
   bias 152
   criticisms 152–4
   ethical issues 147–8
   interpretation 145–8
   methods 65–6, 143
   note-taking 144–5
   validity 147, 149–52
open-ended questions 12, 92–3, 114, 130–1
opportunistic sampling 87
ordinal data 94–5

Index

participant observation 140
perception 136
phenomenology 10–11, 58
photographs 65–6
pilot study 17, 30, 101–2, 126
placebo 32–3
population 33
post-test only designs 42
postal surveys 82, 102–5
potency 29–30
pre-coding 93, 115
pre-test post-test designs 41–2
presentation, qualitative research 73–4
privacy 147
probes 119, 122
prompts 119, 122
purposive sampling 15

qualitative research 7–8, 26, 55–76
    data analysis 17, 68–73, 105–6, 129–30
    data collection 17–18, 62–6
    data handling 66–8
    designs 58–62
    presentation 73–4
quantitative research 7–8, 55
    see also measurement
    data 18, 128–9
quasi-experiments 44
questionnaires 12, 13, 82–3
    design 91–102
    postal surveys 102–5
questions
    closed 12, 92
    open-ended 12, 92–3, 114, 130–1
quota sampling 87
quotations 73–4

random sampling 14, 34, 84–5
randomised controlled trials 44–5, 58
ranking, questionnaires 101
rapport 124
readability tests 96, 103
recommendations 19
recording error 121
reductionism 29
reflective comments 124
relationships 9, 45
reliability 27–8, 149–52
reminders 104–5
repeated measures design 38–9

replication 46
reproduction model 152
research
    benefits/limitations 44–7
    conclusions 18–19
    covert 140
    definition 3
    design 8–9, 36–44, 58–62
    methodology 7–19, 136–8
    problem 4–6
    process 3, 5, 19
    qualitative 7–8, 17–18, 26, 55–7
    quantitative 7–8, 18, 55–7
    question 5, 25
resources 91
respondents 119–20
response rates 91, 104
role, observation 143

sample size 89–90
sampling 14–16, 33–4, 84–90
    see also data
sampling frame 84
scales, questionnaires 99–100
semantic differential scale 100
semi-structured interviews 63, 114–15
sense data 136
sequential sampling 15
setting, interviews 113
silences 125
simple random sampling 85
single-subject designs 37–8
standardised interviews 114
statistical tests 9, 106, 128–9
stratified random sampling 85–6
stratified sampling 15, 39
structured interviews 114
subject group designs 38–9
surveys 9–10, 77–111
    see also interviews
    advantages 79–80
    data collection 81–4
    limitations 80
    sampling 84–90
systematic bias 39
systematic error 28
systematic random sampling 85
systematic sampling 15

tape analysis 67, 73
tape-recorders 66
telephone interviews 116
telephone surveys 81–2
themes 70, 73, 129
topic guide 115
training, interviews 113, 118, 123
transcription 66–73, 129–30
transferability 149, 150–1
trend surveys 78–9
triangulation 150

unstructured interviews 63–4, 115

validity 28–9, 45–6
　observation 147, 149–52
　surveys 79
variables 7, 23–4, 27, 30, 42–3
　causal relationships 44–5
　confounding 30, 38
　extraneous 30
verification 28
video recording 65
visual analogue scales 100

within-subject designs 37–9
written descriptions 65